FOREWORD BY JANE FONDA

# YOUR BODY YOUR HEALTH

## How to Ask Questions, Find Answers, and Work with Your Doctor!

# NEIL SHULMAN, M.D.
# ROWENA SOBCZYK, M.D.

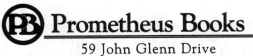

Prometheus Books

59 John Glenn Drive
Amherst, New York 14228-2197

# DISCLAIMER

This book is not intended to substitute for the medical advice of a physician. The reader should regularly consult a physician about matters relating to his or her health and particularly regarding any symptoms that may require medical attention.

Published 2002 by Prometheus Books

Inquiries should be addressed to
Prometheus Books
59 John Glenn Drive
Amherst, New York 14228–2197
VOICE: 716–691–0133, ext. 207
FAX: 716–564–2711
WWW.PROMETHEUSBOOKS.COM

06 05 04 03 02    5 4 3 2 1

Library of Congress Cataloging-in-Publication Data

Shulman, Neil.
    Your body, your health : how to ask questions, find answers, and work with your doctor! / Neil Shulman, Rowena Sobcyzk ; foreword by Jane Fonda.
        p. cm.
    Includes bibliographical references and index.
    ISBN 1–59102–012–3 (alk. paper)
        1. Medicine, Popular. 2. Physician and patient. 3. Self-care, Health.
I. Sobcyzk, Rowena, 1948– II. Title.

RC81 .S49 2002
610–dc21

2002068111

Printed in the United States of America on acid-free paper

Doctor! Doctor!
Stitch me up!
Here's my body;
Fix it up!

I'll close my eyes
And play along;
Just cure me, heal me,
And don't take long!

Zoe Haugo

## FURTHER PRAISE FOR
## *YOUR BODY, YOUR HEALTH*

"This book can significantly reduce the number of malpractice cases. ... [I]t will open new lines of communication between doctors and patients."

–Ronald A. Karp, former president,
Trial Lawyers Association of Metropolitan Washington, D.C.

"In this age of risk management where you must take charge of your own health, *Your Body, Your Health* emerges as the must-read manual for empowering yourself in your interactions with the health-care system, making the system work for you, and feeling good about pursuing good health."

–Kimberly M. Thompson, associate professor of risk analysis
and decision science, Harvard School of Public health,
and author of *Overkill*

"This book will be a comprehensive compass for the consumer–to help [with] navigation through the U.S. health-care systems. ... Drs. Shulman and Sobczyk are to be congratulated ..."

–Mary Starke Harper, Ph.D., RN, FAAN, D.Sc., LLD,
member of the National Advisory Council,
National Institutes of Health

This book is dedicated to my children, Emily and Fred, and all children, in the hope they will listen to their mom and have a long, healthy life.

Rowena Sobczyk, M.D.

I was blessed with a famiy who cared about family, friends, and the community. Israel (dad), Mary (mom), and Larry and Stan (brothers) created a wonderful environment for me so I could grow up and be healthy. Love was the underlying theme. Thanks "y'all."

Neil Shulman, M.D.

# CONTENTS

# CHAPTER 5.  HOW TO AVOID ILLNESS (WASH YOUR HANDS BEFORE . . .)                   135

# CHAPTER 6.  UNDERSTANDING YOUR MEDICAL TEST RESULTS (MED SCHOOL 101) 167

# ACKNOWLEDGMENTS

Many thanks go out to our families, friends, and colleagues who offered their enthusiastic support and suggestions throughout the entire writing process. Special thanks to our editor, Linda Greenspan Regan, for her guidance, gentle manner, and ability to get two stubborn doctors to agree about text. Bill Grabe, thank you for plowing through early versions and pointing out areas in need of clarification. Dr. Kenneth Braunstein, thank you for sharing your expertise in the field of hematology. Elizabeth Vance (emvance@bellsouth.net), our graphic designer, you did a wonderful job of creating understandable illustrations. Patient Care Technologies and Mark Braunstein, we thank you for all the technical assistance and advice you provided regardless of the time of day. Special mention goes to Emily Braunstein for having the vision and courage to suggest major movements of text although the book was in its final stages. We know these suggestions greatly enhanced the readability of the book.

Many diagrams in this book are modifications of those which come from the book *Let's Play Doctor* (ISBN 0-15-503620-3), available from Rx Humor, 2272 Vistamont Drive, Decatur, Georgia 30033, telephone (404) 321-0126, fax (404) 633-9198, nshulman@bellsouth. net, Web site: www.dochollywood.com.

# FOREWORD

by JANE FONDA

**D**on't just show your body to the doctor and ask what's wrong. For the best heath care, it's important to be a partner with your doctor when seeking treatment. You already know more about your body than anyone else does, since you are with it twenty-four hours a day. Exercise, nutrition, clean water, low stress, positive thinking, and creativity are all essential ingredients for keeping your body healthy. However, even living a healthy lifestyle does not guarantee good health. We are all susceptible to illness and we all need to be medically screened for early detection of health problems. The bottom line is that good communication with your doctor is essential.

We are truly at the dawn of a new era in healthcare. The traditional view of the physician as all-knowing is giving way to the concept of the patient and the physician working together as a team to prevent as well as control disease. Patients are increasingly viewing old age as a continuation of life and are looking for ways to remain healthy, vibrant, and involved well into the nineties. I know I am!

There has been a dramatic revolution in the healthcare industry over the last century. Gone are the days of the lengthy house call by the doctor who is knowledgeable in all areas of medicine. The knowledge base of medicine has expanded at a mind-boggling pace. It's as though each individual word in a single book has multiplied into encyclopedias requiring thousands of libraries just to house them. About fifty years ago, the first antibiotic was discovered, and now there are thousands of approaches available for detecting, evaluating, isolating, growing, and stamping out germs. The war on cancer alone has created a highly trained army of specialists. Just keeping up to date on the evaluation and treatment of one rare type of cancer often requires a lifetime of research and clinical practice by an international team of medical subspecialists.

As a result of this knowledge explosion, doctors are busier, evaluations and treatments are often more expensive, and patients are at a higher risk of suffering from complications of therapy. Unfortunately, mistakes cause around 100,000 patient deaths in American hospitals every year. If we want to benefit rather than suffer from this tidal wave of medical advancements, then we, ourselves, must become medically literate. We need to be empowered with knowledge in order to proactively help our doctors help us. The first step toward living a long and enjoyable life is maintaining a healthy lifestyle. The next step is learning how to be a partner with your doctor. This book is a tool to help you take that second crucial step!

# INTRODUCTION

Typically, after sitting for hours in the waiting room, you get literally only two minutes of face-to-face time with your doctor. How do you make the most of it? Empower yourself by gaining critical medical knowledge that will enable you to be in partnership with your doctor and to make smart healthcare decisions for yourself and your family. Be prepared for your visit. Learn how a doctor thinks. Know what doctors look for. Understand what diseases are likely for your age group and gender. Be able to interpret and request basic medical tests. Be aware of recommended preventive and screening services that your doctor should be ordering and know when you need them. Take care of your body by learning how lifestyle impacts your health. This book will give you the information to demystify the basics of a medical visit and be your guide to controlling your health and the decisions that are made about your body. It will give you the necessary medical knowledge to monitor your health with a clinical perspective.

This book can be viewed as "user's guide" for getting good healthcare and an "owner's manual" for your body. The first chapters look at the mechanics of an office visit and then the book moves on to discuss the leading causes of death for various age groups and preventive health measures that can make a difference. The later chapters deal with more technical information and can serve as a reference tool for the interpretation of commonly ordered medical tests and medical terminology. Included is a guide to using the Internet to seek out medical information or to research the latest medical advances that may benefit your health. Each chapter ends with Empowerment Tips. These are reminders of what you can do to forge a partnership with your doctor and take charge of your own health.

**Chapter 1** details the typical office visit, and includes a description of what occurs on a daily basis during an average doctor visit. It takes you from the frustration of being put on "terminal hold" by the receptionist, to getting an appointment, and then through the actual visit and examination by the doctor. Along the way, you will learn to efficiently schedule an appointment and get more out of every visit.

**Chapter 2,** "How Doctors Make a Diagnosis," explains how a doctor reaches a medical conclusion about your health status. You will be able to see the medical visit from the point of view of the doctor. You will gain a greater understanding of the tools available to physicians: the medical history, the physical examination, and medical testing. You will learn how to prepare a concise summary of relevant symptoms related to your problems that your doctor will actually listen to. The importance of making sure the doctor is aware of your genetic background, prior illnesses, and current medications and/or supplements is emphasized. You will realize what areas of the body the doctor should examine and be empowered enough to point out physical changes and abnormalities.

**Chapter 3** discusses how you can start getting more than just standard medical advice out of a visit to your doctor. You will learn to go to every visit prepared to participate in decisions about your health. You will understand the benefits and rights you have under your health insurance plan, and you will learn to avoid treatment delays by having all the necessary forms with you. Finally, you will gain knowledge so you can question a treatment plan and decide if a second opinion is appropriate. Although questions to ask about any medication prescribed are discussed, specific disease treatment is not covered.

The start of your body's "owner's manual" is really **chapter 4**. Knowing what may kill you and when will alert you to symptoms you might otherwise ignore. Starting from infancy and going through old age, you will learn about commonly occurring diseases that require medical attention. Based on your symptoms, age, and gender, you will understand what diseases are likely. You will learn when it is absolutely important to go to the doctor and what should be tested for at every stage of life. Hopefully, seeing the statistics in black and white will give you the incentive to be proactive about your health.

An ounce of prevention is still worth a pound of cure. In **chapter 5** you will explore the basics of caring for your body and promoting longevity, from simple hand washing to recommended preventive healthcare services and screening. You will learn what you can do, on a daily basis, to promote better health. You can't ward off every illness, but you can at least give your body a fighting chance!

Unfortunately your body does not come with a diagnostic chip, so sometimes multiple testing and retesting is necessary to figure the source of illness. Your doctor says you have high good cholesterol. What does this mean? **Chapter 6** will demystify common medical test results. It will explain in plain language what various test terms mean and what area of the body is being tested. It will teach you how to interpret commonly ordered medical tests and procedures. In addition, you will learn why medical testing is not perfect and why simply retesting may be the next best step.

The Internet is leading the healthcare information revolution. Vast amounts of medical material are available to anyone with a computer and Internet access. **Chapter 7** will demonstrate how to evaluate a healthcare Web site and find accurate health information on the Web. Use this knowledge in partnership with your doctor and make informed decisions about the medical care that is best for you or your loved ones.

Frequently used medical words, terms, and phrases are explained in the **glossary**. You don't need an advanced college degree to understand what's happening in healthcare. These are not strict dictionary definitions, but ones that show common usage geared to improve your communication with your doctor. Every chapter can also be used as a quick reference guide for the empowered healthcare consumer.

# CHAPTER I

# THE TYPICAL OFFICE VISIT

## (Ugh! I Must See My Doctor Today)

I t's Monday morning and you're feeling terrible. You call your doctor and the line is busy. Three hours later, when you finally get through, the receptionist places you on hold before you can even get in a word. You memorize the entire Muzak tape before she comes back and, after hearing your request to be seen by the doctor, informs you that no appointments are available. After much pleading, she agrees to squeeze you in three days later. You arrive early for your appointment only to wait thirty minutes before anyone is even aware of your presence. Another hour or two passes as you thumb through old *People* magazines. Finally, a nurse puts you in an exam room. While freezing in just a paper gown, you wait some more. Eventually your doctor breezes in, takes a quick look at you, hands you a prescription, and is gone before you can collect your thoughts. *It doesn't have to be this way!*

Learning how to efficiently get an appointment with the right doctor is the first step toward empowering yourself to be in partnership with your doctor. This is the vital first step in making healthcare decisions that affect your body and your health. To do this, you need to know the type and qualifications of the doctor you should see.

Then figure out the appropriate kind of appointment to request and understand how your doctor's office actually schedules them. Your goal is to decrease time lost while calling the office, lag time until your appointment, and time spent waiting in the waiting and exam rooms. To achieve these goals, the Monday morning scenario you just read will be revisited and experienced through the eyes of an empowered healthcare consumer. You will discover what to do when no appointments are available and then learn the secrets for getting more out of every visit. Vital signs, laboratory tests, and even talking to your doctor will take on new meaning.

Before picking up the telephone and trying to make that appointment, consider what kind of doctor you should see and what kind of appointment you need. A primary care physician can treat common everyday problems, handle many emergencies, and care for chronic conditions. Specialists, as the name implies, specialize in a particular field of medicine such as neurology, neonatology, or psychiatry. They will treat only medical problems that fall into their narrowly focused area of medicine. These days, most primary care physicians are also specialists. They specialize in the basic everyday medical problems most people encounter sometime during their lifetime. The public tends to use the term "specialist" for all fields of medicine other than those which involve primary care. In actuality, any physician who successfully completes a residency program after graduating from medical school is a medical specialist in the field of his or her residency program. In addition, if the physician then passes a certifying examination and continues to meet standards set by the particular specialty, he or she is board certified in that field of medicine. For example, a doctor who, after medical school graduation, goes on to successfully complete three years studying in a family medicine residency program is a specialist in family practice. When this same physician passes the certifying exam given by the American Board of Family Practice, he or she is a board certified specialist in the field of family medicine. To remain certified, the physician will have to successfully complete a certifying exam every seven years and meet continuing medical education requirements.

It is possible to practice medicine without undergoing the additional training of a residency program and without being board certified. This kind of doctor is known as a general practitioner. Many managed healthcare plans insist that their doctors be both residency trained and board certified. To find out more about the various specialty fields of medicine or to see if your doctor is a specialist and is board certified contact the American Board of Medical Specialties at http://www.abms.org on the Web or by phone at 866-ASK-ABMS (866-275-2267).

No matter the specialty or board certification, to practice medicine legally a doctor must be licensed by the state in which the office is located. A healthcare consumer living in another state can be seen by that doctor but he or she has to go to the doctor's office. If the doctor wanted to make a house call on a patient living in a different state, he would also have to be licensed to practice medicine by the state where the patient lives. Each state has its own laws regarding the practice of medicine, and professional standards a doctor must follow to maintain licensure. When a physician does not adhere to the laws or the standards, a disciplinary action is taken by the state against the physician. This can be a fine, a practice restriction, or a permanent loss of licensure. As part of the licensing procedure all states verify the educational background of the physician requesting a license. They require that the applicant has passed a rigorous examination testing medical knowledge and skills, they review disciplinary actions from other states, and they consider any past arrests and convictions. The purpose of this is to protect the healthcare consumer from fraudulent practices and unprofessional medical conduct. To find out more about the rules regarding the practice of medicine in your state, contact its regulating body or visit the Web site of the Federation of State Medical Boards at http://www.fsmb.org. To find out where your doctor is licensed to practice medicine and if any disciplinary actions have been filed against him or her, go to the Web site sponsored by the Federation of State Medical Boards at http://www.docinfo.org.

Most medical organizations consider general practitioners, family practitioners, pediatricians, and internists as primary care doctors because they coordinate your healthcare among different doctors and settings. Some medical organizations also include obstetricians and gynecologists in the primary care designation. Pediatricians care for healthcare consumers from birth to about age sixteen. Internists typically see only adult patients. Family practitioners are trained to care for people of all ages and many still deliver babies. Obstetricians and gynecologists see only women patients for conditions involving the reproductive organs. The type of patient seen by a general practitioner varies from practice to practice depending upon on the interest and skills of the individual doctor.

Any good primary care doctor will refer you to the appropriate specialist as the need arises. In general, fees for a primary care visit are less than a specialty visit so unless you believe that you need a specialist, from an economic standpoint, you are better off seeing your primary care doctor. In the past, health maintenance organizations (HMOs) and other health plans did not allow direct patient access to specialists in an attempt to limit healthcare costs; you had to be referred by your primary care physician. Hence, the term "gate keeper" was developed to describe the role of the primary care physician. However, as they have been able to negotiate discounted fees from specialists, many HMOs and health plans now allow self-referral. This, however, can lead to overuse of specialists by patients. As a result, sometimes it can be very difficult to get an appointment with a specialist when you really need it.

Thus, you may want to consider going to your primary care physician in this situation because she can arrange for you to be seen sooner by the specialist and may even call the specialist to get advice on starting a therapy while you are waiting for your appointment. When treatment is initiated, your visit to the specialist is really a follow-up visit. The visit to the primary care physician will have saved you the higher cost associated with one visit to the specialist. In the case where the primary care physician does not initiate treatment, often the office fee will be waived. For example, you have a prolapsed hemorrhoid, an extremely painful condition. Your primary care doctor takes a look and arranges for you to see a surgeon that day. He may not charge you for the visit because the surgeon will be providing your treatment. Not all doctors will do this, so you do run the risk of paying for an extra visit. You have to decide if getting your problem cared for sooner is worth the potential extra cost. Keep in mind that, even if the professional fee is waived, you still may be responsible for a co-payment, depending upon your type of health insurance. This is particularly true with HMOs that employ physicians. The administration of this kind of HMO typically doesn't give their salaried physicians the right to waive a co-payment. If you want your co-payment waived, you will have to talk to someone in administration, not the doctor.

Having determined the type of doctor you would like to see, it's time to figure out what type of appointment you need. Basically there are three types of appointments, assuming your doctor isn't one of the few practices that work on a first come, first served basis. A routine appointment is one that can be scheduled at both the patient's and the doctor's convenience. This appointment category includes scheduling for things like management of an on-going medical condition, general physical exams, and Pap smears. If this appointment is delayed for a week or two, it probably will not impact your health. A follow-up appointment is one requested by your doctor. It needs to be scheduled within the time frame the doctor recommended. Usually follow-up appointments are made during the check-out process prior to leaving the doctor's office. Sometimes the doctor will make the follow-up appointment optional. You will be directed to come back within a set time frame if your symptoms have not improved or if you are getting sicker. It is very important that you let the receptionist know that the doctor instructed you to be seen for follow-up. This obligates the receptionist to check with the nurse or doctor if your request can't be accommodated in a timely manner. The third type of an appointment is for acute or urgent care. Most offices leave room in their schedules for these appointments. The scheduling dilemma for the office is to predict accurately how many acute care slots are needed on a given day within a given week and still have room for all the routine and follow-up appointments. Ideally, you should be able to get an appointment for an acute problem on the day it occurs.

However, some problems are more acute than others. You need to use some judgment deciding how quickly you need to be seen. For example, a changing mole does not have to be seen immediately but should be seen within a week. If the receptionist does not have any acute appointments available within a reasonable amount of time, *request a call back from the nurse or doctor* to discuss your problem. If you are told that you can't get an appointment for two or three months, then request that the doctor or nurse call you back to verify it is okay to wait that long. There is no point arguing with the receptionist. This person usually does not have any medical training and can't be expected to evaluate the seriousness of your problem. Make sure the receptionist reads your message back to you. *If your doctor thinks that you can safely wait for two or three months, this opinion will now be part of your medical record.* Faced with your concern, the receptionist will often just squeeze you into the schedule or immediately transfer you to the nurse for further evaluation of your problem. If not, when your doctor or nurse calls back, she should give you an appropriate appointment based on your symptoms. You can ask to be placed on a waiting list, but depending upon the efficiency of the office, you may not be called even if a cancellation occurs. Consequently, if you want to get in sooner for a problem, you need to call back on a daily basis and ask about cancellations.

Large health maintenance organizations have a patient services department. If you are having trouble getting an appointment, make sure you call this department and lodge a complaint. In most cases the patient service representative will be able to help you. In response to patient complaints about delays in getting appointments, Kaiser Permanente, a large and well-known HMO, has gone to a same-day appointment scheduling system at many of their facilities. Many other HMOs, health plans, and large practices are following this trend. With same-day appointments, you can get an appointment the day you call and you can also schedule routine appointments in advance.

Mondays and Fridays are typically the busiest days for a doctor's office because of the weekend. People who fall ill over the weekend want to be seen on Monday and those who become ill during the week want to be seen before the office closes on Friday. Many practices also close early on Fridays for religious and other reasons. In addition, many planned procedures or tests requiring a short recovery period are scheduled on Fridays to decrease the amount of time lost from work. The day before and the day after major holidays are busy for similar reasons. Unless you are prepared to wait for a long time, avoid calling the office or scheduling a routine appointment on these days.

The middle of an office session is the best time to call. You avoid the "first thing in the morning" and "last minute" callers. For example, if the office is open from 9:00 to 12:00 in the morning and from 1:00 to 5:00 in the afternoon, the best times to call would be around 10:30 in the morning and around 3:00 in the afternoon. Even better is if your doctor has a Web site that allows you to schedule an appointment on-line. If your doctor does not have such a Web site, you might want to mention to the receptionist that you feel a Web site would benefit your doctor's practice. Keep in mind that at the turn of the century doctors were slow to accept the use of telephones as a means of advising and treating patients instead of having to make a house call. Pressure from patients helps speed the acceptance of change.

Before you try to schedule that appointment, you also need to be aware of your doctor's office scheduling routine so you can plan accordingly. When is the office open? Are limited hours available on the weekend? When is the office closed for holidays and vacations? Can you make a same-day appointment? How far in advance do you need to call to schedule a routine appointment? For example, if your child needs a physical exam to attend summer camp and it takes a month to get a physical appointment, call by May or earlier. If you wait until June to call, camp may be over before your child can be seen. You may want to mark your appointment calendar with when you need to call so that routine preventive visits to the doctor don't get postponed or forgotten.

At the time of scheduling, be candid and ask the receptionist if your appointment is the time you can expect to see the doctor or just the time you should arrive at the office. Many offices build time into the scheduling process to cover filling out insurance and other forms. Find out if there is any advantage to arriving early. You are only increasing your wait time if you arrive early for an appointment and the doctor is not expected until fifteen minutes after your arrival. However, if the office schedules more than one patient per appointment slot, even if extra time is allowed for forms, the person who arrives early for that slot will be seen first. This is known as wave scheduling. It is common in big cities since it takes into account the variability of traffic as well as people's habits. Wave scheduling assumes one person will come early, one on time, and one late. You want to be the early one so you don't have to wait for the doctor to finish with the other two people.

You also need to know your doctor's schedule. If your doctor has hospitalized patients, when does he visit or "make rounds" to see these patients? Ideally, you want the doctor's first appointment of the morning or afternoon when rounds aren't being made. In this way you are seen before the doctor starts running late. Rounds can take longer than the time allotted depending upon the severity of illness of the patients hospitalized. Similarly, any given patient can take longer than planned, so you want to be the first.

Illnesses and accidents occur at all hours. You need to know your doctor's policy and your health insurance coverage for the delivery of after hours and emergency care. In the case of a life- or limb-threatening event, go to the nearest emergency room. By law, all health plans have to cover the use of the nearest emergency room for true life- or limb-threatening emergencies. For everything else, you will need to use some judgment because if you go to the nearest emergency room for less than a "true" emergency, your health plan may not pay for or may only partially reimburse your visit. A medical emergency means that failure to get immediate medical care could put a person's life in danger or cause serious harm to a person's bodily functions. Some examples of a medical emergency include, but are not limited to, an apparent heart attack, uncontrollable bleeding, sudden loss of consciousness, and severe injuries. The emergency room is a very expensive place to receive healthcare so it is smart to call your doctor before going—but only if your health will not be affected! At the very least, your doctor's office will have a message telling you where to go for care after hours or will give you a number to call for advice. If you do not have a regular doctor and you need emergency advice, many hospitals have triage or advice lines that you can call to see if an emergency room visit is warranted. However, they will not be able to give you information about what your health insurance plan will cover. In addition, before you go you might want to consult a quick reference book on emergency symptoms.

You now know the type of doctor to see, the kind of appointment you need, and the best time to schedule it, so it's time to return to Monday morning. Remember, you are really sick. You call mid-morning and the receptionist picks up on the third ring. She informs you that your doctor has no appointments left and does not offer you an appointment with another doctor or other healthcare provider within the group. Ask to speak to the nurse. Tell the receptionist that you will hold for the nurse. In the situation where you need a same-day acute appointment, you do not want to be called back. You need to work on other arrangements for healthcare if the nurse can't help you with your illness or work you into the doctor's schedule. You are very polite and calmly describe your illness but the nurse has no medical advice to offer about your illness and will not give you an appointment with anyone in the practice. Do not get angry. The nurse is following office protocol and will be more likely to help you if you remain pleasant. Ask to speak to your doctor. The nurse refuses to let you speak with your doctor. She will only give your message to the doctor. Leave one but don't expect a prompt response.

Assuming you don't get called back and your illness is severe and you decide not to seek healthcare elsewhere, you still have an option. Doctor's offices do not like it, but you can always just walk in without an appointment. Make arrangements to arrive at the office thirty to forty minutes before it closes for lunch. If you are lucky, you will get squeezed in before the lunch break. If not, you will most likely be seen early in the afternoon session. *No office likes to have an obviously ill patient sitting for hours in the waiting room.* If your doctor is part of a group practice, a different provider within the group may see you. By walking in without an appointment, you give up your right to choose which provider in the office will see you. Your actions demonstrate to the medical office that you are too sick to wait for an appointment. In this situation, you want to be seen as quickly as possible. Although you may prefer a particular doctor, there is no reason to think that another provider can't at least stabilize your condition until your regular doctor is available.

Your persistence plays off and the nurse arranges for you to get an appointment later in the day. Sick as a dog, you still manage to arrive a few minutes early for your appointment. No one is at the front desk or no one seems to be aware that you are in the waiting room. Don't grab the nearest *People* magazine and sit. Go to the front desk and get someone's attention. Deliberately dropping the clipboard with the sign-in sheet usually will get someone's attention without causing any damage. Be prepared to produce your insurance card, picture identification, social security number, payment method, and any referral or visit authorization forms and medical records needed for the visit. If you are bringing someone else's child to the doctor, you'll need a signed "Authorization to Treat a Minor" consent form or other authorization if you aren't the parent or legal guardian. A child you are babysitting, even if you are a relative such as a grandparent, is not legally allowed to be seen and receive treatment from *any* doctor without the authorization of a parent or guardian unless it's a life- or limb-threatening emergency. A simple note from the parent giving you permission to authorize treatment on the child, or the consent form, is all that the doctor will need.

Failure to have the required paperwork will increase your waiting time. You will not be allowed to see the doctor until it is available. Double check with the receptionist when you make your appointment to guarantee you will have all the forms and records you will need for the visit. The office will not tie up an exam room while waiting for needed information to arrive by fax or phone. You will be sitting in the waiting room until whatever is missing arrives, or you may be asked to reschedule your appointment if it becomes apparent that the material can't be readily obtained.

No office can guarantee that you will be seen in a timely manner. Real emergencies do arise, so always bring something to read or do while waiting. If you bring a laptop computer, make sure your battery is fully charged, since an electrical outlet may not be available. Once you have waited for fifteen minutes, ask the receptionist about the delay. Depending upon her answer, you may want to reschedule. Doctor's offices are notorious for long waits. In a well run office you will voluntarily be given some sort of explanation and/or apology after waiting for more than fifteen minutes. Computer software exists that allows physicians to schedule their practice efficiently. As an empowered healthcare consumer you need to let the office staff know that your time is valuable. Offices have no incentive to make scheduling changes unless healthcare consumers speak up. Some offices will notify you of appointment delays if you give contact information, such as your cell phone number, at the time you make your appointment. Alternatively, call before you leave for your appointment to make sure the doctor is still running on time. In fairness, you should notify the office if you will be more than fifteen minutes late and cancel any appointments you know you can't keep.

Finally, a nurse appears and calls out something close to your name. You follow the nurse to the scale. Shoes really don't weigh that much, but go ahead and take them off if it makes you feel better. Weight is relative so try to be weighed the same way every visit. Your doctor is looking for trends in your weight. Is your weight stable or are you gaining or losing weight? What's important is whether you weigh too much or too little for your height, age, and gender. Your doctor will have no documentation of the trend of your weight unless it is taken at every visit. Because a doctor can visually estimate whether you are over- or underweight, she may not realize the nurse has failed to take your weight until the trend is needed. Then it is too late. Your weight today can provide valuable information about your health in the future so ask to be weighed no matter how emotionally painful it is. If a change in your weight is unexpected, mention this to your doctor.

Depending upon the reason for your visit, some laboratory specimens may now be obtained. If you are directed to leave a urine sample in a cup, make sure your correct name or other form of identification is placed on the cup prior to depositing a sample. If a label is not already on the cup you will need to write your name on it. A full cup is not necessary. When done, put the cup on the specimen shelf in the bathroom unless directed otherwise. For blood tests, offer the finger or arm that you prefer be used. The index finger of your dominant hand does not have to be sacrificed. Tell the person taking your blood sample when you last ate. Food can interfere with the results of certain blood tests. If you believe the doctor will be ordering additional blood samples for a number of tests, mention this to the nurse to avoid being stuck twice. Also mention any other tests that you are interested in having performed. Pregnancy tests, blood sugar levels, and tests for strep throat are good examples. Some offices allow the nurse to obtain certain tests at the request of the patient so that the results are ready when you see the doctor. This can save you the time of being sent back to the laboratory and waiting for the results.

Not all tests that are routinely ordered are always necessary. Dr. George Lundberg, the former editor of the prestigious *Journal of the American Medical Association*, wrote a book about the problems of our healthcare system, *Severed Trust: Why American Medicine Has Not Been Fixed.* He states in this book, "about 80 percent of the tests carried out in the laboratories I oversaw in academic medical centers did not need to be done."[1] Ask why you are being tested. If you are not given a good reason, refuse to be tested until you have discussed the test with your doctor. A common example of routine testing currently not recommended by the United States Preventive Services Task Force (USPSTF) and the American College of Obstetricians and Gynecologists (ACOG) are the urinalysis and the hemoglobin blood test healthy adult women with normal menstrual periods get ordered during their Pap smear visit. Testing when it is not necessary only increases the cost of healthcare without yielding a reasonable positive return. In other words, the risk and cost associated with the testing is greater than any healthcare benefit you might receive. (USPSTF is made up of doctors from all disciplines of medicine who carefully review scientific evidence about tests and other preventive health measures and determine what actually results in improved health outcomes. ACOG performs similar work but is made up only of doctors specializing in obstetrics and gynecology.)

Make sure the results of all tests are discussed with you. Often you are never given the results of your tests even though they are placed on your chart for the doctor. You can ask for a copy of the results. Most offices won't charge you for copying a laboratory test result. It is nice to have your own record of certain tests so you can track improvement in your health such as decreasing blood fat levels. Your office visit may take a little longer but you will be starting to participate in your own healthcare management.

Vital signs are usually taken next. They reflect the overall pattern of your health. Most doctors will agree that your blood pressure and your pulse should be measured at every visit. Many will also measure how fast you breathe and your body temperature. These measurements are very easy and painless to obtain. However it is important for them to be obtained correctly. If you have just finished a hot or icy cold beverage tell the nurse since this could affect an oral temperature reading. The normal temperature for an adult is anywhere from 97.5° to 99.6°F, depending upon the time of day and ambient room temperature. Remove your arm from your shirt for the most accurate blood pressure measurement. This can be tricky if you are in a hallway and not the exam room. However, rolled up sleeves can restrict blood flow and cause an incorrect reading. The lower portion of your arm should be horizontal and supported at the mid chest level. If the cuff placed on your arm is below the level of your heart when your blood pressure is measured, erroneously high pressures can result. If you have a large arm, a larger cuff may need to be used. A blood pressure cuff that is too narrow can also cause incorrectly high readings. The blood pressure cuff should be wide enough to cover 80 percent of your upper arm and rest about half an inch to an inch above your elbow. A small cuff is used to take blood pressure in children and very small adults. Remind the nurse about a smaller or larger cuff if that is the way your blood pressure is usually taken. Incidentally, the nurse can't hear you with the stethoscope in his or her ears. Talking can cause a higher reading so be silent during this part of the examination but don't hold your breath. Proper cuff alignment is pictured in figure 1.

You are taken to the exam room and the nurse asks the reason for your visit. State your problem as plainly as possible. By understanding your problem, the nurse is able to make sure necessary supplies and equipment are in the exam room prior to the doctor's arrival. This makes for a more efficient visit with the doctor. The doctor will then not have to leave the room or ask for an assistant to

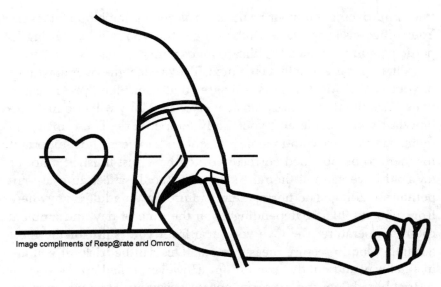

Image compliments of Resp@rate and Omron

## Figure 1. Proper Blood Pressure Cuff Alignment

bring something in after you have been placed in a compromising position. Volunteer to the nurse any allergies that you have, either to medicines or any other substances. This information must be in your medical chart. Your doctor may need to change routine diagnostic testing and medication orders because of your allergies. Also tell the nurse about any medications–prescription, over-the-counter, herbal, or otherwise–that you take or have taken recently. Any of these products may be contributing to your current health problem.

Supposedly, the thin sheet of paper the nurse hands you protects your modesty. Take off all clothing as directed and wrap up as best you can. Ask for an extra drape if you find the room is cold. Access to your naked body makes it easier for your doctor to figure out what is wrong with you. Abnormal heart and breath sounds are much harder to hear through tee shirts or slips and your doctor should be able to look for abnormal moles and other skin problems you may not have noticed. After the nurse leaves, the doctor should arrive shortly. If the wait in the exam room exceeds fifteen minutes, stick your head out the exam door and politely remind the nurse that you are waiting.

Sometimes a doctor accidentally sees patients out of order or simply forgets that someone is waiting in a particular exam room.

The doctor arrives. According to the January 2001 Harris Interactive survey, you now have *two minutes of face-to-face time* with him or her. Since this poll reflects the average on any visit you may get more time than that, especially if you need a complete physical examination or have a very complex problem. On the other hand, with a simple common problem you may get less. In any case, you want to make the most of the time you get. Describe your problem. "Make me well" does not provide any clues to help your doctor solve your problem and gives up any control you have over your own healthcare. If you are worried about a certain diagnosis or disease, immediately express your concern. Don't operate under the assumption that if it's serious enough the doctor will find it, whether you say something or not. It is helpful to have a list of your medical concerns. With a prepared list your thoughts are organized and you can quickly mention everything. Be sure to mention your biggest concern and/or main symptoms first. If you wait until the doctor's hand is on the exam room door ready to leave, chances are your main fear or symptom will not be seriously addressed or you will be told to make another appointment to address that issue. For example, you are embarrassed by your dandruff but also have athlete's foot. Don't wait until the doctor has already written a prescription for your athlete's foot and is leaving to mention the dandruff. If you mention it then, you might just be advised to use an over-the-counter shampoo and to schedule another appointment if that isn't successful. You want a serious evaluation and, if necessary, a prescription for a hair product on that first visit.

The doctor asks a few questions about your problem and then examines your body. Unless you are there for a complete physical exam, the examination is usually limited to the area of the body affected by your problem. For example, if you have an ear ache, you can expect the doctor to examine your head, neck, and possibly your lungs. If you have a stomach ache, expect the doctor to exam your abdominal area and possibly do a rectal exam. (See figure 2, "The Abdomen.") With a complete physical exam, the doctor should

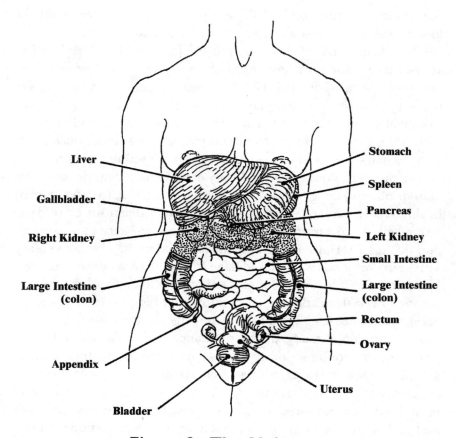

## Figure 2. The Abdomen

illustration by Elizabeth Vance, adapted from Rx Humor (www.dochollywood.com)

examine every part of your body. This includes all orifices or openings. Women should expect a pelvic and rectal exam and men should expect a prostate and testicular exam. Patients hate the rectal exam. However, it is an important part of a physical. In addition to looking for abnormalities such as hemorrhoids, during the rectal exam a doctor can examine the backside of the uterus and ovaries in women and the prostate gland in men.

After the examination, the doctor may order tests. Make sure you understand what is being ordered, why it is being ordered, and where you need to go to be tested. Find out when you can expect the results and how you can get them. Should you call for the results? Will the office call you? Do you need to make a follow-up appointment? If you give permission, can the results be left on your home answering machine? Can the doctor send you a secure e-mail message? If the doctor does not have a secure e-mail messaging system, you might ask him to send a nonspecific message by e-mail or voice mail that your test results are normal. Remember, no news may not be good news. Just because you have not heard from your doctor does not mean your test result was normal. Test results get misfiled and lost both at the laboratory and at the doctor's office. Make sure you get all your test results. It would be a shame to delay early treatment of a serious illness such as cancer because a test result was not reported.

It turns out that you have a minor illness that does not require further testing but will need to be treated with a prescription drug. Do you want a prescription for a generic medication? Generic medications are usually equivalent to brand name medications but less costly. Unless your doctor has a reason for requesting the brand name medication, you should get the generic. In addition to being less costly, a generic prescription is easier to fill. The pharmacist can dispense any equivalent medication currently stocked by the pharmacy. This can avoid ordering delays if the pharmacy does not stock the brand of medication your doctor prescribed. Almost every managed healthcare plan has a formulary, a list of prescription drugs, both brand name and generic, that your health plan has agreed to cover. Medications not on the formulary will probably cost you more. Check with your health plan. Many plans now have Web sites that list your alternative drug options and drug information or will send you a copy of the formulary so that you can be in partnership with your doctor to decide the best prescription choice for you. Whenever your doctor needs to write a prescription, it is up to you to remind her about the formulary of your plan. Don't end up spending more than necessary for medications.

It is late in the day and you are afraid that your pharmacy will close before you can get there. Ask the doctor if this will cause a problem. Doctors expect their patients to start taking medication the day it is prescribed. Often your doctor will be able to give you a free sample of the medication if you can't purchase it immediately. In addition, your doctor may have a coupon from the manufacturer of the medication that will offer you savings. Qualified patients can get certain medications for free, so if you can't afford your medications make sure to tell that to your doctor.

You get a sample of your medication so you can immediately start treating your medical problem or condition. Your doctor says it may cause mild nausea. This is a known side effect, not an allergic or adverse reaction. Side effects are generally less serious than allergic or adverse reactions. If the side effect is mild, you will be expected to continue taking the medication. Sometimes just changing the time of day you take your medication by twelve hours can eliminate a side effect. Ask if a given time of day is better than another to take the medication. Your doctor should discuss the main side effects and bad reactions your medication can cause so you know what to expect when you take it. Remind him of all other medications, herbals, and supplements you are taking to avoid drug interactions. As the use of herbals has become more common, the list of their known interactions with prescription medications is rapidly growing. Interactions can be serious. They occur when one medication reacts with another. For example, certain antibiotics interact with birth control pills, making the birth control pills less effective in preventing pregnancy. When you fill your prescription, your pharmacist should also provide you with drug interaction and side effect counseling. If you use more than one pharmacy, make sure they know all the drugs you are taking.

If you have a bad reaction to the medication or are not sure about your reaction to it, don't take another dose. This is important, as some serious reactions that appear mild with the first dose get much worse with the second dose. Contact your doctor or pharmacist immediately for further advice. Your pharmacist may be easier to contact than your doctor and is an excellent resource for information about drugs and drug reactions. In addition, your pharmacist will speak directly with your doctor about your reaction when medically necessary. It is possible for a serious medical allergy to develop at any time during the course of treatment, not just after the first or second dose. Even if you have taken the medicine before or have been taking it for several days, you should stop the medication and call for advice if you have a bad reaction. You also need to find out from your doctor how long it will take before the medicine starts to help relieve your symptoms or improve your health.

Whether you have a minor ailment or a major disease, you need to find out whether or not your illness is contagious. Can you inadvertently pass this disease on to someone else? Do you need to take any preventive measures beyond the usual of not sharing food, beverages, or towels? How much medication do you need to take or what needs to happen before you are no longer contagious? For example, twenty-four hours must pass from the time you begin taking the antibiotic for strep throat before you are able to go back to school or work to ensure you are no longer contagious. Think about your daily schedule. Is it okay for you to return to work or school? If not, how long should you plan on being absent? Do you have any physical restrictions? You may not feel like jogging five miles, but is it okay to modify your exercise program so you don't get out of the habit? Move on to your weekly calendar. Do you have anything planned that your illness may prevent or that may require special precautions? For example, you have a sinus infection and need to fly on business. Your doctor may want you to take a prescription decongestant prior to boarding.

As the doctor leaves, you are told to come back in three days if you aren't feeling better. It is important that you understand from your doctor what to expect about the course of your illness. You need to know what occurrences would cause the doctor to want to see you again. For example, a week ago your doctor gave you a prescription-strength decongestant because you had a bad cold. You still are congested, just started coughing up green sputum, and your chest hurts. Do you just continue taking the decongestant? As a general rule, anytime you have been seen for an illness and new symptoms develop or old symptoms get worse instead of better, you should recontact your doctor for additional advice. Depending upon the severity of your symptoms, schedule a follow-up appointment, ask to speak to the nurse, or leave a message including your new symptoms and requesting a call back that day.

Your doctor hands you a sheet of paper called an Encounter Form for the billing desk and then leaves the exam room. After getting dressed you may leave the paper "drapes" for the nurse to discard, or throw them in the trash yourself. Do not put drapes or other trash in the red cans that are marked biohazard. Form in hand, you finally find the billing desk. You hand the Encounter Form to the clerk and are asked for payment. Most doctors expect payment at the time of service. If you can't pay the whole amount, now is the time to make arrangements for a payment schedule. If you have insurance, you will be charged your plan's co-payment. A co-payment is the small part of the physician's fee that the healthcare consumer is expected to pay. The purpose of a co-payment is to help keep healthcare premiums lower so more employees can afford the cost of buying coverage. Employers and insurance companies use co-payments to pass some of the cost of insurance on to the members who receive healthcare benefits. Less healthy employees and those with larger families use more healthcare services, yet their healthcare premium is the same as that of the married employee who rarely gets sick or has only one dependent.

The first step in becoming an empowered healthcare consumer is to determine the best type of doctor to consult for a visit and then efficiently schedule an appointment whether it is for a routine, a follow-up, or an acute care appointment. Bring all pertinent documents to the scheduled visit so that care is not delayed. During the visit, make sure vital signs are properly checked, all concerns and symptoms are discussed with the doctor, and any advice and treatment plan is explained. Take an active part in the visit, voicing all medical concerns and giving specific and clear answers to the doctor's questions. Allow only necessary tests to be performed and obtain all results. Most importantly, start acting in partnership with your healthcare provider to make informed healthcare decisions.

There is no question that our healthcare system needs improvement. Do your part to bring about change. Through empowerment, you can start to receive the quality care you deserve. This sentiment is also echoed by Dr. George Lundberg: "Complete patient and family participation in decisions about patient care are among the critical changes that must be made to mend our broken system."[2]

# EMPOWERMENT TIPS

▼ Call mid morning or mid afternoon.

▼ Schedule routine appointments well ahead of time.

▼ Make sure your need for an "acute" appointment is known.

▼ Have necessary documents available at time of check-in.

▼ Express your main concerns early.

▼ Make sure vital signs are taken correctly.

▼ Understand the reason for all tests.

▼ Understand your treatment plan.

▼ Get all your test results.

▼ Don't overpay for medications.

# CHAPTER 2

# HOW DOCTORS MAKE A DIAGNOSIS

## (Think Like a Doc)

Now that you're aware of how to get an appointment and what to look out for during a typical office visit, it's time to look at that visit from the doctor's point of view. Imagine you are the doctor. If you understand what the doctor is trying to accomplish, you can make sure nothing important gets overlooked and truly take charge of your health. More detailed information on previously introduced topics will be given to increase your ability to meaningfully communicate with your doctor.

Most of the time, the doctor can figure out what is wrong with you by listening to what you say about your illness. The details about your current problem combined with the rest of your medical history are the most important clues the doctor has to make a diagnosis. Pay close attention to what your body is telling you so that you can fully and accurately describe your symptoms to your doctor. Sir William Osler, one of the most influential teachers of physicians in history, is quoted as saying to young doctors, "Listen to the patient and he will give you the answer." In other words, hearing from you the symptoms that are a departure from your normal state of health starts the doctor's deductive reasoning process which results in your diagnosis.

By the way, if you are in for just a routine examination such as a Pap smear visit or an employment physical and have not experienced any unusual symptoms, use your time with the doctor to go over any questions you might have about your health in general.

The anxiety you feel about being sick and about how a serious illness would affect your life colors the way you present your history to your doctor. Because of this, you need to focus on the facts when you are giving your history. It is important to mention what you are afraid of so the doctor will address the issue. However, fears do not supply your doctor with any diagnostic clues. Through your words, you want to give your doctor the clearest possible picture of what is going on with your body. Talk about all your symptoms without lessening or exaggerating them. Keep in mind that just because a doctor does not ask about a particular symptom does not mean the symptom isn't important. Doctors are not mind readers and they don't always remember to ask all the questions they should. A study published by Dr. P. G. Ramsey in the *American Journal of Medicine* showed that primary care doctors failed to ask important medical questions 59 percent of the time.[1] Consequently, the second step to being an empowered healthcare consumer is to report all your symptoms, even if you feel they are meaningless or fear what they might mean. Use whatever words you feel comfortable with to describe your problem. You do not have to use medical terms. Your doctor will ask for clarification if he does not understand your meaning. If you can't speak for yourself because of a language barrier or disability, bring someone along who can accurately describe your problem and answer additional questions. In situations where you are very upset or not sure what happened, it is helpful to bring along a family member or friend for emotional support and to provide supplemental history. In the case of an accident or other trauma, a witness to the event or a written report of the event, such as a police report, can often supply useful information to the doctor. For example, you are involved in a fender bender and walk away from the accident. The next day you see your doctor with severe back pain. The police report can help the doctor understand the kind of forces your body was subjected to and provides an objective accounting of what happened. A Volkswagen

Beetle has less impact than a SUV, so your doctor needs to know which of these hit your car.

Identical symptoms can produce greatly different diagnoses from the same doctor. Your speaking pattern and appearance also provide valuable information. The ability to speak a whole sentence without gasping in pain or gulping air gives your doctor some basic information about the intensity of your illness. Sitting upright with a smile on your face as you say your stomach hurts will get a different reaction from your doctor than if you say your stomach hurts while bent over clutching your abdominal area. Likewise, if you hop up onto the exam table wearing skintight blue jeans, your doctor will not believe that you are experiencing incapacitating lower back pain. Your doctor evaluates how you look as well as what you say in making a diagnosis.

Although it is important to *tell your doctor all of your symptoms*, you do not have to give every detail of your day. Your doctor will get impatient and redirect you if your history includes too much extraneous material. Sometimes valuable information gets lost because of this. You need to give your doctor a concise listing of your symptoms. Let your doctor ask you for the more specific details. For example, tell your doctor that you have had a sore throat for two days and that it is getting progressively worse. He does not need to know that you first noticed your sore throat at 10:00 at night before you could floss and brush your teeth and put your children to bed.

Your medical history is separated into three distinct parts: the history of your present illness, the history of your past illnesses, and the history of illnesses that run in your family. You will be questioned in each of these areas as each can impact your current illness and your health. Your doctor may not always go over your past medical history or your family history if all this information is available on your chart and you have a simple medical problem. Nonetheless, doctors don't always read the chart thoroughly and may not remember your case so speak up if you feel your history is pertinent. If you are being seen for a complete physical examination the doctor should go over all three parts of your medical history. Even if you aren't asked, if you have seen a different doctor for a serious illness or if someone in your family has developed a new disease since your last visit, be sure to update your doctor. The information you provide may be a valuable clue to your current problem and/or could signal your doctor to recommend a preventive health measure.

## HISTORY OF PRESENT ILLNESS

When giving the history of your present illness, you need to tell your doctor some basic information about this departure from your normal state of health. First give the anatomic location of your problem. Follow this with a complete description of the problem, starting with how the problem began and ending with your current symptoms. Discussing your symptoms is like being a reporter. Your doctor needs to know the whole scoop—who, what, where, when, and why. To illustrate, let's assume you have a stomach ache. The who is the area of concern: your stomach. The what is the pain. The where is in the right lower side of your stomach (see figure 3 to help locate your pain). The when is constantly for the last four hours. The why will be determined with further evaluation by your doctor in partnership with you.

The more information you provide your doctor, the easier it will be to figure out the source of your problem. How long have you had the problem and is it getting better or worse? Think about factors that irritate or relieve it. What makes your problem worse? What makes your problem better? Some problems occur only in certain physical positions. What have you tried for relief? Heat and ice are commonly used to give relief of symptoms. Have you taken any recent trips or participated in an activity that may be the source of the problem? Contaminated water associated with travel and camping is a common cause of illness. Unusual physical activity may be a source of the problem. Many people see the doctor for lower back pain a day or two after moving heavy furniture. How intense is your problem? Is it severe enough to keep you from sleeping at night? Does it keep you from performing your job or going to school? Does it bother you only at certain times of the day or during certain activ-

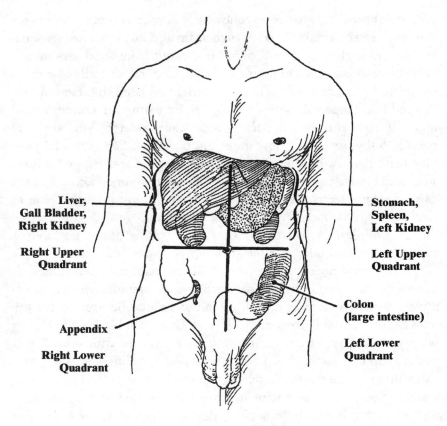

## Figure 3. Locate Your Pain

illustration by Elizabeth Vance, adapted from Rx Humor (www.dochollywood.com)

ities? Describe the nature of the problem. This is especially true when talking about pain. *Stabbing, sharp, dull, tearing, crushing,* and *burning* are good, descriptive words to use. How did the problem start? Did it come on gradually or all of a sudden? Where were you when the problem started? The environment at the onset may be contributing to the problem. If you get a headache when you visit your neighbors, perhaps their pet cats are the cause. Have you ever had the same or a similar problem? Do you also get a headache when you go to the pet store? Does this problem tend to run in your family? All your brothers are allergic to cats, so maybe that headache is related to your neighbors' cats. Does anyone else you're in contact with have a similar illness? Certain illnesses such as flu and hay fever are seasonal and others such as food poisoning can result from food served at a party or restaurant. All of us are aware of the recent recalls of ground meat from grocery stores. The government recalled the meat to prevent additional people from getting sick by eating the contaminated meat. If your problem is accident- or injury-related, you also will need to tell your doctor how the event occurred. For example, your foot twisted inward while you were running or you tripped over a stool and landed on your outstretched arm. Sometimes, show and tell can be very effective. Seeing the bug that bit you or being able to read the ingredients off a product label will help your doctor narrow the possibilities. If you think something that is easily portable is causing or contributing to your problem, bring it with you.

Your doctor needs to know about all medications, prescription or otherwise, that you currently are taking. This includes vitamins, laxatives, herbal remedies, and other supplements. Be able to list the name, amount, and frequency. If you have trouble remembering what you take, make a list and bring it with you to your visit. If you prefer, you can just put all your medication containers in a bag and show them to the doctor. Especially in the case of prescription medication, don't let your doctor assume you are taking it as she prescribed if that is not the case. You doctor needs to know if you are doubling up or skipping doses. You may be damaging your health if you don't confess. Be honest with your doctor and tell him how you're really taking the prescribed medication and why. Based on your reason, it is possible that your doctor can either change the medication or the dosing schedule to one that is more acceptable. Also, what you are taking and how you are taking it may be affecting or even causing your current illness.

Sometimes your doctor will need to ask additional questions about your present illness. Through this questioning process, the doctor is starting to form a list of possible causes for your illness and is starting to solve the riddle of diagnosing your illness. The list is known as your differential diagnosis. The doctor will use the rest of your history, findings from your physical examination, and results from tests and procedures to confirm or rule out the diagnoses on this list. For example, you complain of sudden onset of tiredness, nasal drainage, nasal obstruction, sneezing, and coughing which all started one day ago. Based on just this history of your present illness, your differential diagnosis includes the common cold, nasal irritation from allergies, nasal irritation from an environmental source, or a more serious infection.

## PAST MEDICAL HISTORY

Your lifestyle is part of your past as well as your present medical history since things you did in the past could affect you now. Lifestyle typically refers to your exercise habits, nutrition, sexual practices, smoking, and drug and alcohol use. It also includes job hazards and other exposures. Your current and past lifestyle can make you more or less susceptible to specific diseases. As you get older, things you did or did not do when you were younger may come back to haunt you. Recent studies have shown that regular exercise in your teen years lowers your risk for breast cancer.[2] On the other hand, a history of smoking increases your risk of lung disease. If you have developed a good or bad habit make sure you mention this to your doctor. Your doctor will have helpful tips about your new good habits such as a regular exercise program and may be able to help you stop the bad ones such as smoking. Understandably you may find discussing your present and previous bad health habits with your doctor difficult and embarrassing, but your doctor really needs to know about them. Illegal drug use, high-risk sexual behaviors, and sexual difficulties are probably the most awkward problems for healthcare consumers to talk or even hint about to their doctor. Another lifestyle issue that is extremely difficult to discuss is domestic violence and suspected child abuse. Believe it or not, your doctor really is there to help, not to judge. Many resources are available to help in these situations and your doctor is a great way to start finding them. *Remember, what you tell your doctor is confidential. Legally, your medical record can't be released without your permission.*

Life events are also part of both your past and present medical history. A life event is any important happening or change in your life, good or bad. Not surprisingly, life events play a major role in your health. It has been known for a long time that married men live longer than their single counterparts. They may not have more fun, but they do live longer. Interestingly, a high number of life events occurring close together will increase your chance of becoming ill, even if all the events are *positive*! Your doctor should be informed of major life events such as a new job, marriage, extramarital affair, or divorce to determine if the life event is impacting your current illness or if any preventative measures need to be taken to help protect your health. For example, you have some mild stomach pain and have had an ulcer in the past. Knowing you have a new job, your doctor may choose to start you on a stronger ulcer medication than over-the-counter antacids to prevent a reoccurrence. A new job is stressful, although the adjustment time varies from person to person and with the job. Because of your past history, your doctor is now aware that, in response to stress in the past, you developed an ulcer. You are at higher risk of developing an ulcer in this new job situation than a person who has never had an ulcer. This will be taken into consideration when deciding the most appropriate treatment for your current stomach pain. In addition, your doctor may want to test you for the bacterium *Helicobacter pylori* if you had not been previously tested. It is now known that ulcers can be caused by the presence of this organism and the treatment is an antibiotic regimen to kill the bacteria present in the intestinal tract.

In relating the rest of your past medical history to your doctor, try to recall all significant medical events that have occurred. These include previous serious illnesses, surgeries, and significant physical exam findings. Your doctor should help jog your memory by asking things like, "have you ever had trouble with your heart or been told you have a heart murmur?" Be sure to mention all chronic diseases you've suffered from, even if the disease has not been active for years. For example, if your mother said you had asthma as a child (sometimes also called reactive airway disease), mention that to your doctor. Gestational diabetes, or high blood sugar levels when you were pregnant, is another example of an inactive past medical problem that your doctor needs to know about. Certain past diseases may be more or less relevant depending upon your current state of health. You can expect more detailed questioning from your doctor if a past disease is considered important. *As a rule of thumb, any past illness affecting the same part of the body as your current illness should be mentioned.*

## FAMILY HISTORY

The rest of your medical history is your family history. Your doctor takes your family history into consideration in the process of forming your differential diagnosis. It's not easy to escape your genetic background. Certain diseases run in some families. In some cases the responsible gene is known and can be traced and tested for. Genetic testing can be used to predict your likelihood of developing a disease. In addition, you can be advised on your chances of passing a particular disease on to your child before you get pregnant. Table 1 lists some common illnesses in which family history plays a role.

Great strides are currently being made in the field of medical genetics that will probably benefit all of our lives. Even if your family history has no relevance to your current problem, it can provide you and your doctor with a list of diseases to watch out for. This does not mean nothing can be done or that you will definitely get a particular disease. Knowing you have a higher than normal chance or are at risk for getting a disease because it runs in your family can change the way you receive healthcare. Your doctor may initiate screening tests at an earlier age or at more frequent intervals to catch the disease at an early, more curable, or more easily treatable stage. Your doctor may suggest preventative measures to stave off the illness. For example, if high blood pressure runs in your family, as a preventative measure your doctor might encourage you to have a regular exercise program, limit the amount of salt in your diet, and to watch your weight.

Consequently, think about what has happened to your relatives and immediate family members since your last visit. If someone has

---

## TABLE 1. COMMON ILLNESSES IN WHICH FAMILY HISTORY PLAYS A ROLE

▼ Cancer—especially breast, colon, prostate, and ovarian

▼ High blood pressure

▼ Diabetes mellitus—especially non-insulin dependent

▼ High blood fat levels

▼ Alcoholism

▼ Mental illness

▼ Autoimmune diseases—those where your body attacks itself

▼ Domestic violence and child abuse

---

passed away, make sure you know the cause of death, age at death, and if it was a maternal or paternal relative. Just knowing your favorite uncle died recently is not enough. You need to be able to report that your maternal uncle died of a massive heart attack at age fifty-six. Remember, your lifestyle, life events, and family history are an important part of your overall health and need to be updated every visit. As an empowered healthcare patient you need to understand the relationship between your family history and your health.

## PHYSICAL EXAMINATION FOR PHYSICAL SIGNS OF ILLNESS

After discussing your present, past, and family history, your doctor usually has a good idea about the cause of your medical problem. He or she will now perform a physical examination to look for the actual physical signs that go along with that illness. (A brief overview of what an exam entails is provided in table 2.) The change your illness produces in a specific part of your body is a physical sign. A physical change is usually definitive and obvious. Your doctor can objectively

## TABLE 2.  BRIEF OVERVIEW OF A COMPLETE PHYSICAL EXAM

| Body Part | Specific Areas Usually Examined |
|---|---|
| General appearance | Obvious abnormalities, distress, hygiene, level of consciousness, how you walk, speech, body stature |
| Head | Skull, hair, scalp, face, sinuses |
| Eyes | Ability to see; eyebrows, eyelids, tear ducts, external eye; internal eye is examined with by a hand-held ophthalmoscope |
| Ears | Ability to hear; external ear; ear canal and tympanic membrane are examined with a hand-held otoscope |
| Nose | Internal nasal mucosa and passages |
| Oral Pharynx | Lips, gums, teeth, tongue, palate, throat, tonsils |
| Neck | Lymph nodes, thyroid gland, trachea, carotid artery, jugular vein |
| Chest | Prior to listening to your lungs with the stethoscope, the chest wall may be palpated and tapped, breasts examined |
| Cardiovascular system | Pulse and the heart felt and the stethoscope used to listen for abnormalities |
| Abdomen | Organs are palpated and tapped and the stethoscope used to listen for abnormalities |
| Male Genitalia | Lymph nodes, hernias, scrotum, penis, testicles |
| Female Genitalia | Lymph nodes, hernias, internal examination both manual and with speculum |
| Rectal exam | Anal opening, a digital exam is done internally to feel for abnormalities |
| Musculoskeletal system | Muscles, joints, tendons |
| Neurological system | Level of consciousness, cognitive abilities, muscle strength and coordination, reflexes, sensation, individual nerves are examined |
| Skin | Texture, scars, swelling, other abnormalities |

see the signs of your illness as opposed to hearing you subjectively relate your symptoms. Typically, your doctor will examine the part of your body that is primarily affected by the problem you mentioned and nearby areas. If you feel your doctor is looking at an unrelated body part, you might ask him why. This is an opportunity to increase your medical knowledge about how the various parts of the body interact. It can also serve as a deterrent to unprofessional physicians who abuse the privilege of being a doctor and examine certain body parts unnecessarily. To lessen this concern, most male physicians will only examine a female patient with a nurse or other medical staff member present in the room.

## DIAGNOSTIC TESTING AND PROCEDURES

Based on your history and the findings of the physical exam, your doctor now has a pretty clear idea of what's wrong with your body. To be certain of what's going on, additional testing may be needed. Diagnostic testing and/or procedures may be done in the office or you may have to go elsewhere to obtain them. Sometimes health problems are so complicated that you have to undergo a battery of tests before the diagnosis can be made. This can be very frustrating and you may wonder why all the tests couldn't have been ordered all at once. Unfortunately this is not always possible. Tests need to be performed in a certain order, as the result of one test may lead the doctor down a different direction for the next test. Undergoing all possible tests at the same time can cause over-testing. You may prefer to get it all over with, but a shotgun approach to testing is not in the best interest of your health. Any diagnostic test can potentially cause harm. For example, in the unlikely case you have an allergic reaction to the contrast material used, certain X-rays can make you very ill and even kill you. Your doctor has to carefully weigh the benefits of a test over the risks to your health.

Your doctor also keeps your medical costs to a minimum by ordering only the tests that are needed to make your diagnosis. Some healthcare consumers request screening tests that are not recommended for the public at large. Most health insurance plans will not pay for these tests. You may want a particular test, but just because a diagnostic test is available does not mean that you need it from a medical point of view. For example, many women want to get a CEA 125 blood test to check for ovarian cancer at the time they go in for a routine Pap smear. This test, however, is not recommended as a screening test for ovarian cancer by any respected medical organization. Your health plan will pay for the pelvic exam that accompanies a Pap smear visit but will probably not pay for a CEA 125 blood level unless other indications are present. This does not mean that you can't get a CEA 125 test. You can still request and receive any test your doctor agrees to order as long as you are willing to pay for it. (On the horizon is a new blood test for ovarian cancer that shows promise as a screening test for this deadly disease, but it is currently not generally available.)

Depending upon what is ordered and when it can be scheduled, you may not learn your final diagnosis on the first office visit. However, your doctor should discuss his concerns and what he suspects is wrong with you so you know why the further testing is necessary and what he hopes to learn from it. If you are a nervous type of individual who always assumes the worst, just ask your doctor outright what the worst likely diagnosis could be.

## TREATMENT PLAN

Having taken your history, examined you, and reviewed the results of all ordered tests and procedures, your doctor now has several options based upon whether a diagnosis was made, whether one can be made soon, and whether your doctor feels she can help you. One of the common options is to treat your problem with medications. This may consist of prescription medication or you may be advised to purchase a nonprescription or over-the-counter medication such as a fever reducer or antacid. Antibiotics are not effective in the treatment of common everyday illness such as colds and sore throats that are caused by a virus. *Antibiotics don't work against viruses, period!*

Taking antibiotics when they are not needed helps bacteria develop resistance to them. As a result, an antibiotic may not work when you really need it. A few antiviral medications do exist, but their use is restricted to certain diseases. Your illness may not need any medication but instead may require supportive treatment and time to heal on its own. Your doctor will describe the supportive treatment methods he wants you to use. Common supportive treatments include bed rest, increased fluid intake, ice packs, heating pads, and even the fabled chicken soup.

When possible, your doctor will fix your problem then and there. This usually involves a manipulation or application to the affected body part. The wax will be removed from your ear. Your laceration will be sewed, stapled, or glued together. A cast or ace bandage will be applied. Make sure you understand what your doctor is going to do, what result you can expect, and what steps you need to take afterwards. If you are not sure this is the best treatment option for you and delaying treatment will not further harm your health, you may want to ask for a second opinion.

In certain cases your doctor may feel that another doctor or specialist is better suited to care for your medical problem. In these instances, your doctor will probably recommend a particular doctor or type of doctor for you to see. Make sure you understand who is responsible for setting up the referral appointment. Will your doctor's office make the appointment or do you need to call? Depending on your health insurance, your choice of specialists may be restricted. It is wise to ask your doctor for a recommendation because your doctor may feel a certain specialist is better than others. Even if your doctor makes the appointment, make sure you have any required referral forms and are provided with the necessary medical information to take to the referring doctor. For example, you may need to take pertinent X-rays and lab test results with you.

Sometimes the best treatment option is to do nothing. Your doctor may tell you that he wants to wait and see what happens. Perhaps your disease is stable right now and does not need treatment yet or may go away on its own. Or it might be that your doctor doesn't believe that your problem is of any consequence and will disappear with time. If your doctor is not clear about what is going on, she may wait to see what other symptoms develop in order to make an accurate diagnosis. In this situation make sure you clearly understand when to schedule a follow-up visit. If you are not comfortable with waiting, you may want to seek a second opinion to put your mind at rest.

You may have an unusual, very complicated, or rare problem. In this situation your doctor may need to find out more information in order to provide you with the best possible treatment options. Your doctor will ask you for time to do some research. Since medicine is changing so rapidly, it is impossible for your doctor to stay current on everything. Consequently, this is a very reasonable request. Where your doctor needs to go to get more medical information about your problem will determine how quickly he can get back to you. Have a clear understanding with your doctor as to *when* you might expect an answer and how you will receive the information. Do you need to make a follow-up appointment? Do you need to call the office? Will you be called or get a secure e-mail message? Also, find out if there is anything you should be doing while waiting to hear back.

Although most doctors take as much time with you as your medical situation warrants, clear communication encourages good rapport. If you logically, accurately, and concisely describe the history or your present illness and update your past and family medical histories without prompting, more time may be spent going over your treatment plan and any questions you might have as a result of your diagnosis. Your doctor wants you to follow his advice and can help you take charge of your health. It is up to you to lead the way, so don't just turn your body over to the doctor and say "go to it."

# EMPOWERMENT TIPS

▼ Prioritize and describe all your symptoms.

▼ Don't add unimportant details.

▼ Be honest about your lifestyle and habits.

▼ Mention all medications and supplements.

▼ Discuss your family history.

▼ Mention major life events.

▼ Understand your treatment options.

# CHAPTER 3

# HOW TO WORK WITH YOUR DOCTOR

## (Do Your Homework)

To get more out of your office visit than just standard medical advice and warnings requires a change in mindset. Too many people worry only about what they are going to wear to the doctor's office, not how they are going to use the doctor to get answers to improve their health. Hippocrates (460–370 B.C.E.), the father of medicine, developed the principles of medical diagnosis and treatment along with a code of ethics for medical care. Most doctors are ethical, but not all possess a friendly bedside manner. You should feel comfortable talking to your doctor. Some doctors will label patients they don't get along with, because of personality clashes, as "difficult." They may treat their "difficult" patients with less regard and try to pass their healthcare onto other providers within the organization. This is known as dumping. If you feel you are being dumped from one provider to another within a group, or if you leave every appointment feeling rushed and uncertain with unanswered questions and concerns, consider changing to a doctor with a different bedside manner or a to different group. Remember, your doctor has to believe that you are sick. If you have a doctor who believes your illness is "in your head," you will not get effective treatment or good advice.

## YOUR DOCTOR IS A CONSULTANT

You need to start thinking of your doctor as your personal healthcare consultant instead of as the person who can make you well. Your body, not the doctor, makes you well and keeps you well. Together with your doctor, you can do things to maintain health and to speed the healing process, but it is up to your body to remain healthy and to recover. Obviously, you know your body better than anyone else. You are the person who must do the preventive maintenance to stay well and who experiences the symptoms of illness when disease strikes. Consequently, it is common sense for you to be in partnership with your doctor in making healthcare decisions.

Think about how you work with other consultants in your daily life. You state the problem, answer any additional questions the consultant might have, and then you discuss the report that the consultant prepares. Throughout the entire process, you are in control. It is up to the consultant to present compelling reasons for you to follow his advice. In other words, start relating to your doctor in the same way you relate to your auto mechanic. Prior to taking your vehicle in for service, you list the performance issues you have with the vehicle and, in addition, any preventive maintenance tasks you want performed. Unfortunately your body does not come with an owner's manual. The mechanic will discuss the performance issues, look at your vehicle, and then discuss your options and the cost of each. Based on this, you decide whether or not you want the work done. If you are not sure about what the mechanic recommends, you talk to a knowledgeable friend or see another mechanic. Start relating to your doctor in this fashion. Don't be intimidated. The doctor is the consultant and you are paying to hear and understand his medical opinion of your problem.

Just as being friendly with the mechanic helps you get better vehicle service, having an ongoing relationship with your doctor is an advantage. A doctor who understands how you reacted to illness in the past can put your current symptoms into proper perspective. In addition, she can tailor your treatment to your preferences. For example, if you have religious beliefs that preclude certain treatments, your doctor may be able to advise acceptable alternatives. Within your health plan, your doctor is your advocate. Obviously a doctor who has a long-standing relationship with you is more likely to fill out forms and to petition committees to help you get the care you want. This help can be as simple as obtaining a brand name medication instead of a generic or as complex as getting a surgery approved for coverage. If your doctor says something is not allowed by your health insurance plan, make sure you ask about how an appeal can be filed. The practice of medicine is not always clear cut. Through an appeal, your case will be reviewed by a different doctor or panel of healthcare providers who may feel an exception to the health plan protocol is warranted in your case. During the appeal process, the medical reasons why an exception should or should not be made in your case are discussed. As with everything else in life, it never hurts to ask.

## KNOW YOUR COVERAGE

Needless to say, healthcare delivery is more critical for you than getting your vehicle serviced because it involves life and death. Although you can always buy a new car, you only get one body. In addition, healthcare is complicated by health insurance and health plans. Vehicular service and repairs are either under warranty or they are not. You pay for work not covered by warranty, so you decide what gets done, when, and where. Depending upon what kind of healthcare insurance you have, your choice of healthcare providers may be limited, the insurance payment for a service may be less than the doctor bills, or you may not even be allowed to have a certain service covered. Part of preparing for your doctor visit is figuring out if your problem is covered by your insurance and, if it is, which type of doctor you may consult. Your insurance card is imprinted with telephone numbers and information to help you with this process. If you have never looked at your card, it is wise to read the information on it prior to seeing your doctor so you know the basics of your healthcare coverage. A complete listing of your benefits can be found in the brochure you received from your insurance carrier or on their Web site. Unfortunately, this information is often confusing. Discuss what

you don't understand with your employer's human resource department or contact your insurance carrier's customer service department.
Typically, you will need to know the social security number of the
health insurance policy holder and the group identification number in
order for the customer service representative to answer your questions. The latter can be found on your insurance card.

Health insurance basically comes in two forms: traditional, fee-for-
service or indemnity plans and managed care plans. As a rule of
thumb, you get greater doctor selection with a traditional plan and
more covered services with a managed care plan. Managed care plans
can be broken down into Health Maintenance Organizations (HMOs),
Preferred Provider Organizations (PPOs), and Point of Service (POS)
plans. With an HMO you are restricted, except in emergencies, to
seeing only doctors within the organization. With a PPO, you pay
more if you don't see a doctor within the organization. With a POS
plan, you get the best outside coverage only if a doctor within the plan
has referred you to the doctor outside the organization. For more information about health insurance and health plans a government Web site
gives in-depth coverage of all the options and what they mean at
http://www.ahcpr.gov/consumer/hlthpln1.htm#choices.

Part of your responsibility when making an appointment is to
find out about typical fees associated with the doctor visit. Also find
out which hospital and outside laboratories your doctor uses to make
sure they are covered by your health insurance. If your doctor is not
on your plan or you do not have health insurance, you want to know
what sort of charges to expect. In addition, although you may choose
to see an out-of-network doctor, you will most likely want to make
sure that she can put you in a covered hospital and order laboratory
tests and procedures from a covered facility, because these services
can be very costly. Don't wait until you are critically ill and in need
of hospitalization to discover you have to change doctors to avoid
paying a larger percentage of your hospital bill. If your doctor has a
Web site, most of this information will be posted on it. Health plans
discourage use out-of-network physicians and facilities because of
cost. For in-network groups, the plan has negotiated a fee for a
healthcare service which is usually less than what the doctor or

facility normally charges, so using an excellent in-network doctor is financially to your advantage. The plan is getting a volume discount. However, under certain circumstances, such as when you are traveling, exceptions are sometimes made to the regular rules.

## HAVE FORMS READY

Obtain and complete your portion of all the forms that you need prior to arriving at your doctor's office. Not having all the information on a form may necessitate an additional visit or a call back to the office. It is best to be prepared. You will be amazed at the amount of information requested that you don't have at your fingertips. This can be anything from the social security number of the health insurance policy holder to the date of your last tetanus shot. In addition, your doctor may not keep the necessary form in his office. For example, you request a handicapped-parking permit to allow you to take a disabled elderly parent shopping. Your parent's doctor will have to certify that your parent is disabled and qualified to receive a handicapped permit. You may need to go to your parent's state motor vehicle bureau first to obtain the necessary form. Similarly, although most primary care physicians have school immunization forms available, double check with the receptionist when you are making your appointment to make sure they are there.

Certain employers and schools require documentation that an absence was health-related. Sometimes just a note from the doctor is not enough. If you need a certain piece of paper signed by your doctor documenting your absence, make sure you bring it with you to avoid the hassles of obtaining a signature later. This is particularly true when dealing with Worker's Compensation and other insurance claims. Not having the paper with you can lead to delays in your case being processed. First your medical chart has to be pulled from the record room. A note has to be made about your request. This will be attached to the form and then given to the doctor for her signature while she is busy with other patients. You can see how the paperwork could be misplaced or continually put off to a less busy day.

# DO YOUR HOMEWORK

Try to gather a little information about your problem so you can utilize your doctor's expertise and be in partnership with him in making healthcare decisions. With the advent of the Internet, finding reliable medical information has become very easy. In the past, only people with access to a medical library could hope to find comprehensive material about their illness. The Internet has changed all that. There are excellent sources of medical information currently available to anyone willing to perform a search. You do not even have to know medical terms to obtain information. Valuable information about many diseases can be found by searching for a symptom or a common name. By reading up on your illness prior to seeing your doctor you will be in a better position to evaluate your diagnostic and treatment options. Of course not all Web sites provide worthwhile information, so be sure to discuss what you have found with your doctor. Even better, print the article and share it with your doctor.

Knowing something about your illness prior to your visit can help you describe your symptoms more clearly. You will be able to focus your mind on the crucial aspects of your complaints and thus increase your ability to express your concerns and have them understood by your doctor. It may also help you to remember or notice an important clue that would have gone unmentioned. As suggested earlier, you may want to create a list of these concerns and bring them with you to the visit. Having some basic medical knowledge provides you with a foundation to request special testing from your doctor when you sense something is wrong. You may be able to recognize subtle symptoms of a disease before they become full-blown. For example a man with the vague complaints of feeling less strong, less interested in sex, and more tired than usual might be dismissed as "working too hard" unless he asks about getting his testosterone level checked. After discussion, the doctor and the man may agree that this is a reasonable suggestion in light of the symptoms and any physical exam findings. Even if the testosterone level comes back normal or if, together, they decide testing is not yet appropriate, the man will have partnered with his doctor in making a healthcare decision. The laboratory results, if obtained, could also lead the doctor in a different, but necessary, direction. Incidentally, if you are worried about your testosterone level, take the "Deficiency in Aging Men" questionnaire located on the Web at http://www.tquiz.com. Use the results to start a discussion with your doctor.

In addition to finding out about the symptoms, testing, and treatment for any problem you are experiencing, you can also learn about disease prevention. You should know if you need to be screened for a specific disease test or to be re-immunized. For example, many adults fail to keep basic immunizations current. Find out the last time you had a tetanus shot. If it has been more than ten years since your last shot, you need a booster. Many adults also fail to get basic screening tests performed like mammograms, Pap smears, and blood cholesterol levels. If a close relative died of colon cancer or a heart attack, you should find out when to request screening. Hopefully your doctor will remind you to get these preventive measures, but as an empowered healthcare consumer you need to make sure nothing is overlooked. It is difficult to request a test that you really don't want to undergo even when you know you need it. The inclination is to feel like you have gotten away with something when your doctor fails to order a needed screening service. However, an ounce of prevention is still worth a pound of cure. Take charge of your healthcare and request from your doctor appropriate screening and preventive measures.

## BE ABLE TO QUESTION A TREATMENT PLAN

Another part of being prepared is to understand the questions that need to be asked about a treatment plan. You don't want to blindly accept advice. Just as you would discuss buying new tires versus just rotating or retreading the old ones, you need to discuss your medical treatment options with your doctor. In the case of any proposed medication, find out if drugs other than the one he is suggesting are available. Ask about the advantages of one drug over another. You want to know why your doctor feels a certain drug is best for your condition. The recent advertising by pharmaceutical companies on television has increased consumer awareness of newer medications. However, just because a drug is new to the market doesn't mean it is the best choice for your current disease. What should you do if you forget to take a dose? How critical is taking the medication at the same time of day? If you start feeling better, can you stop the medication or is it important to continue the regimen and take it all? Do you need to avoid certain foods or alcohol while taking the medication? Would certain foods be helpful? For example, when taking antibiotics, eating live cultured yogurt can decrease side effects because the yogurt replenishes the naturally occurring bacteria within the gut that antibiotics kill. Does the medication require special storage? Some medications need to be stored in the refrigerator or where light can't reach them.

Additionally, you need to discuss what impact the diagnosis and treatment plan will have on your overall health. Not all diseases are treatable, controllable, or curable. In the past, doctors refrained from telling patients they had a terminal illness but the majority of the medical community now recognizes that patients have the right to know. If you have a serious disease, make it clear to your doctor that you want the truth so you can plan your life accordingly. Recognize that no one can tell you exactly how quickly the disease will progress or when it will prove fatal. Many factors determine these things. However, if you have a terminal illness your doctor should be able to tell you the average length of survival from the time of diagnosis. You might want to become an organ donor or sign a living will. It is best if your doctor discusses these important topics with you while you are capable of making such a decision.

When surgery is being considered, you need to focus your questions on the best ways to prepare for the surgery and what to expect during the recovery process. It is a good idea to bring a relative or friend along to take notes for you when surgery is required, because the emotional impact of having to have surgery can make you forget all the advice your doctor is giving you. This is also true when treatment options for any serious illness, such as cancer, are being discussed. Having the notes to read at your leisure will lead to a better understanding of what is planned and can help alleviate some of your unnecessary concerns and anxiety. Always contact your doctor if you have any further questions about a proposed surgery. Your doctor understands that surgery is scary to think about and wants you to feel comfortable.

Traditional medication or surgery may not be the only treatments available. You need to explore the other options with your doctor. The interest and knowledge base in alternative and complementary medicine is growing. Studies have been done that look at the benefits of certain supplements, such as glucosamine for arthritis. When taken properly, glucosamine has be shown to decrease pain and increase movement in people with arthritis and joint pain.[1] Also, medical devices exist that can help in treating specific problems. For example, the use of the medical device RESPeRATE can be an effective supplement to prescription medication in controlling hypertension. Instead of adding another drug to get your pressure down, your doctor may be able to control your blood pressure by having you just breath with this device for fifteen minutes three times a week.[2] (http://www.resperate.com)

## GO OVER YOUR STATEMENT

Remember you are using your doctor as your healthcare consultant. You will be presented with a bill for services rendered. You should go over this statement just like you would any other bill. Even with electronic scanners, the grocery checkout clerk still makes mistakes. Imagine the difficulty the doctor's receptionist has trying to read the doctor's writing. Mistakes do happen. It is up to you to pay attention to what tests and procedures were obtained during your visit so that you can verify your charges. If you feel you are being charged for a service that was not obtained or that the fees are excessive for what you received, discuss the matter with the appropriate office staff member. Bring any statements you question with you from previous visits. It is easier to get charges verified while your chart is pulled from the files and readily available than at other times.

The medical record of your visits to a doctor's office is considered yours. The doctor may keep the original but you have a right to obtain a copy. Legally, your doctor can charge you an administrative handling fee and a copying fee. The maximum fees allowable are regulated by each state. An administrative handling fee of twenty-five dollars plus a copying fee of ten cents per page is fairly standard. On your first visit to a new doctor having a copy of your medical record can be very helpful, especially if you have a complicated medical history. Your new doctor can obtain a copy of your record from a previous doctor or healthcare facility once you have signed the proper release of medical records form, but getting the record can take weeks. If possible, you should obtain a copy of your record and take it with you on the first visit. Ask the new doctor to copy what she needs so that you do not give up your copy.

## CONSIDER A NEW CONSULTANT

Your doctor is your consultant. It is up to the consultant to present compelling reasons for you to follow their advice. Remember you can always get a second opinion. Some insurance companies even suggest you get a second opinion prior to approving certain surgeries. You have only one body, so if you are not sure about the advice that has been given, seek another opinion. Getting a second opinion has become even easier with the Internet. You may not have to travel to see the specialist. Well-respected medical institutions across the country, such as the Cleveland Clinic and Massachusetts General Hospital, have started offering on-line second opinion services. For a fee you can send your medical record for review and second opinion by an expert in the field. However, if you have received a second opinion from multiple well-respected specialists and no one has been able to help you, it may be time for you to focus on other aspects of your life as well as your health.

To get the most out of a doctor's visit, start rethinking how you view your doctor. Begin to assume control of the visit. To that end, you need to be prepared. Fill out your part of any required forms before the visit to avoid delays. Know what healthcare benefits you are eligible to receive before you go. Know what basic screening and preventive measures you need so they aren't forgotten. Be prepared to question any treatment plan and discuss the impact of your diagnosis on your daily life and long term plans. If you disagree with or question what you have been told, request a second opinion. Review all fees and charges before leaving the office. Through preparation you can relate to any doctor as a personal healthcare consultant and empower yourself to work with your doctor in making the best healthcare decisions for you.

## EMPOWERMENT TIPS

▼ Use your doctor as your healthcare consultant.

▼ Read your health insurance card and understand your plan.

▼ Do your health condition homework.

▼ Know what to expect from your illness and treatment.

▼ Go over your bill.

▼ Consider a second opinion.

# CHAPTER 4

# GOOD HEALTH AT EVERY STAGE OF LIFE

## (What to Watch Out For)

None of us is too concerned about getting a common cold or a sporadic stomach virus. Although "sick as a dog" at the time, we expect to make a full recovery. What we fear most are the events we may not recover from. We worry about what will either kill us or drastically change our quality of life or that of a family member. We want to stave off those events whenever possible. According to the United States National Center for Health Statistics, the two leading causes of death are heart disease and cancer, but these diseases don't top the mortality charts until middle age. By knowing at what age a disease is most likely to strike, the healthcare consumer is empowered to start proactive measures. Each stage of life brings new challenges for staying healthy and these challenges are influenced by our gender, ethnicity, and other inherited genes.[1]

## BABIES (JUST BORN AND ALREADY SICK: CONGENITAL ANOMALIES, SIDS)

Of all deaths that occur during the first year of life, most occur during the neonatal period, the first twenty-eight days of life. The greatest number of deaths occur the very first day of life. This makes sense when you consider that, prior to being born, the baby's life functions were being performed for it by the mother through her placenta. After birth, the infant must undergo many physiological and biochemical changes to survive. The lungs must breathe to get oxygen. The stomach has to digest food. The kidneys must eliminate waste materials. The immune system has to ward off infections. If any of these systems fails to start working, the infant will get sick and possibly die. Prenatal care is special medical monitoring and treatment during pregnancy. Mothers who start it in the first three months of pregnancy increase the chances of their baby being born normal and healthy. Although in the United States almost all babies are born in hospitals, not all mothers seek early prenatal care. Medical science has advanced so far that many potential life-threatening conditions can be diagnosed and life-saving interventions made before the baby is born. Surgery can even be performed to correct serious problems while the baby is still in the mother's womb. Early diagnosis is essential, so start prenatal care in the first months of pregnancy.

Home urine pregnancy tests are very accurate if performed by carefully following the instructions on the box. Your doctor uses the same kind of test in her office unless a blood pregnancy test, a quantitative test, is needed to see precisely how much pregnancy hormone is being produced. A blood pregnancy test is used for problem pregnancies. For example, if you start bleeding early in your pregnancy and your doctor is concerned about a miscarriage, he will use a blood pregnancy test to monitor the health of the pregnancy. With a first morning urine sample, a home pregnancy test can turn positive as early as ten days after conception. Thus, there is no excuse not to start prenatal care early in a pregnancy. You need to do what is best for your baby.

## Birth Defects

Congenital anomalies, abnormal conditions or defects that one is born with, are the second most common cause of death up until age four and one of the top five leading causes of death in both boys and girls up to age fifteen.[2] Usually no cause can be found for the defect. However, certain viral illnesses contracted during pregnancy and certain medications, especially when taken early in pregnancy, can cause defects. German measles or Rubella is a common viral illness that can cause birth defects when contracted during pregnancy.

To protect unborn children, many states require women to have Rubella testing or proof of adequate immunization against the disease prior to issuing a marriage license. Of course, this practice will not protect babies born or conceived out of wedlock.

Defects of the heart and the surrounding blood vessels are the most common of all congenital anomalies and occur more frequently in African American babies. The heart develops early in the pregnancy, often before the mother realizes she is pregnant. Consequently, a mother may inadvertently expose her baby to medications and other potentially toxic substances. If you are trying to conceive, avoid alcohol, smoking, and other recreational drugs. Tell your doctor that you are trying to get pregnant so that only medications believed to be safe for the baby will be prescribed.

As soon as possible after birth, your baby should undergo a complete physical examination to look for birth defects. Most mothers instinctively count fingers and toes the first time they hold their baby. Your doctor should carefully examine the baby too. Heart defects are often picked up during a physical exam when the doctor hears a murmur, an abnormal heart sound, with a stethoscope. Heart murmurs are often transient in the first days of life, however, so your baby should be examined again before discharge from the hospital. Heart defects can range from small holes between the chambers of the heart to the heart not being completely formed. The defect can obstruct blood flow in the heart or surrounding vessels or cause blood to flow through the heart in the wrong direction. If your baby turns blue when crying, eating, or moving, mention this to your doctor. Also if you feel your baby has trouble breathing and/or difficulty nursing or taking a bottle, tell your doctor. These may be early signs of heart problems or other congenital anomalies. Your doctor should weigh and chart your baby's growth pattern during the first year of life. Poor weight gain and growth can be a subtle sign of some-

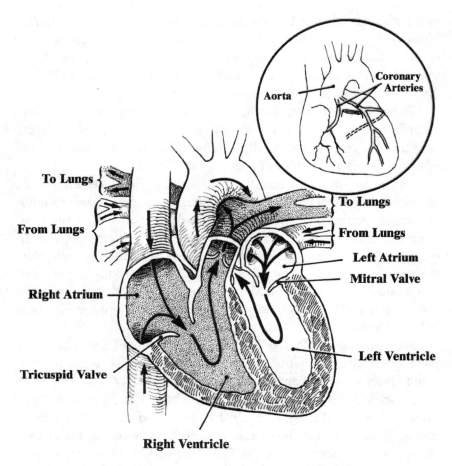

## Figure 4. Anatomy of the Heart

illustration by Elizabeth Vance, adapted from Rx Humor (www.dochollywood.com)

thing wrong. Ask to see your baby's chart. The pattern should reflect a steady increase in growth. Ask your doctor to explain any dips.

Newborns should be screened for more than just physical defects and abnormally developed organs. Abnormalities that affect the body's chemical make-up or metabolism should also be screened for. Typically screening is performed by obtaining a blood sample from the heel of the infant. The federal government mandates this type of neonatal screening. Individual state laws control the exact metabolic screening tests that are offered or are required by the state. All fifty states offer screening for Phenylketonuria and congenital hypothyroidism, which will be discussed shortly. Most screen for hemoglobinopathies, disorders that affect the blood system. Some hospitals offer parents the option of getting supplemental testing done to screen for diseases not required by state laws. In addition, private laboratories will send expectant parents the information to obtain additional testing in cases where a hospital can't provide it. To find out what tests are mandated in your state or to get information about supplemental testing, call the National Newborn Screening and Genetics Research Center at 512-454-6419 or visit them on the Web at http://genes-r-us.uthscsa.edu.

Phenylketonuria (PKU) is a hereditary disease, one that is passed on through families. It results in the body failing to properly break down the common food chemical phenylalanine found in protein. This failure results in severe, irreversible mental retardation unless dietary restrictions are started immediately. With a proper diet, however, retardation can be prevented. If this test is performed during the first twenty-four hours of life, it should be repeated before the baby is two weeks old, as it is more sensitive after the baby has had several meals of either breast milk or formula. With the trend toward early hospital discharge, many babies are screened and discharged before they have had time to eat enough food for the test results to be accurate.

Untreated congenital hypothyroidism, which is more common in baby girls and should be tested for within the first week of life, can also cause irreversible mental retardation. In addition, this disorder causes growth failure. Although affected babies appear perfectly normal at birth, they are born without a functioning thyroid gland. The early symptoms of this condition are subtle and easy to miss, even for a doctor. Testing is the best way to discover the disorder. When diagnosed and treated within the first month of life, the retardation and growth failure can be prevented.

The most common and best-known hemoglobinopathy is sickle cell anemia. Most common in African Americans, the disease can affect all races and both sexes. Your baby needs to be screened for this type of disorder during the neonatal period. Tell your doctor if someone in either parent's family has sickle cell anemia, sickle cell trait, or another form of anemia; this type of blood disorder is frequently inherited. Other, less common, hemoglobinopathies exist and may be tested for, depending upon your state's law.

In addition to PKU and congenital hypothyroidism, other diseases can be screened for by using the same heel prick. Many times parents are not aware of all the screening tests that have been run. They are just told some tests were run to explain the bandage on the baby's heel and are not given any specifics. As an empowered healthcare consumer, you should find out what screening tests you can expect to be performed on your newborn. Request supplemental screening if your state does not mandate screening for diseases you are concerned about. For example, sickle cell anemia screening is currently not required by all states. Idaho, North Dakota, and South Dakota do not require this test. If you live in one of these states and know sickle cell disease runs in your family, request testing.

Make sure your baby receives eye medication shortly after birth. Silver nitrate or erythromycin drops are used to prevent blindness that can occur from a gonorrhea infection acquired during birth from an infected mother. The drops may cause mild eye irritation but this should clear within twenty-four hours. Unfortunately, many women with a gonorrhea infection don't have symptoms and they unwittingly pass the infection on to their newborns. Gonorrhea is a sexually transmitted infection and not all sexual partners, even when they know they are infected, share that they have contracted a "social" disease. A father may choose not to tell his pregnant partner about other sexual relationships, and vice versa. Consequently all newborns should receive treatment to protect their vision. This is done automatically in hospital deliveries, but it is smart to double check. As much as you love and trust your partner, the only sexual behavior you can vouch for is your own.

## Sudden Infant Death Syndrome

Sudden Infant Death Syndrome, more commonly known as SIDS, is a major cause of death for infants between one and twelve months of life. Though it has been killing infants for centuries, the cause of the syndrome is still unknown. Most cases of SIDS occur before six months of age with the peak number of deaths occurring between two to four months of age. More male infants are affected than females. The death occurs quickly during sleep with no apparent suffering. The diagnosis is made only after all other possible causes of death have been ruled out by clinical history, examination of the scene, and autopsy. SIDS is unpredictable and not preventable but several risk factors are known. Sleeping in the prone position (on the stomach), exposure to smoke, and bottle-feeding all increase the chance of SIDS occurring. Consequently, put your baby down to sleep on his or her back, not on the stomach or side. Don't smoke or allow people to smoke around you during pregnancy or around your baby. Choose breastfeeding your infant over bottle-feeding, if at all possible. These behaviors will decrease the chance of your baby dying from SIDS.

## CHILDREN (STILL LITTLE AND SUSCEPTIBLE)

### Cancer

Cancer is the major cause of death from a disease in childhood.[3] Boys are affected more often than girls and there is a higher incidence in Caucasian children. Cancer occurs when cells making up a part of the body start growing and dividing in an uncontrolled manner. The cell growth is disorderly and capable of invading and destroying nearby tissue and organs. These cells may break off and start growing in other parts of the body, thus spreading the cancer. The new cancer that is created by this process is known as a metastatic cancer. Most cancers are named for the type of cell or organ in which they began. For example, breast cancer starts in the breast. Lung cancer that is the result of the spread of cancer from the breast is known as metastatic breast cancer of the lungs.

Although cancer is a leading cause of death in children, with newer treatments many children are cured. If your child is diagnosed with cancer, don't give up hope. Ask your doctor to send you to the closest pediatric cancer center to make sure your child benefits from the most current therapy. These centers are a hospital or unit in a hospital that specializes in the diagnosis and treatment of cancer in children and adolescents. They follow step-by-step guidelines, or protocols, for treatment and offer support programs for the family. To find out more about a pediatric cancer center near you call, or ask your doctor to call, the National Cancer Institute hotline at 800-4-CANCER (800-422-6237).

Childhood cancer differs from adult cancer both in nature and type. The majority of childhood cancers are leukemias, intracranial and central nervous system tumors, and lymphomas. Sarcomas, neuroblastomas, and kidney tumors occur less frequently. Leukemia is a kind of cancer that affects cells located in the bone marrow that are responsible for making blood. Most cases will be of the acute lymphoblastic type. It is called lymphoblastic since too many blood cells of this type are being abnormally made. If your child is unusually pale, persistently lethargic, and doesn't want to eat, ask your doctor to run a simple blood count to make sure leukemia is not present. Intracranial tumors and tumors involving the central nervous system are those located in the head, brain, or spinal cord. Frequent headaches and morning vomiting can be a symptom of this kind of cancer. Lymphoma is a cancer that arises in the lymph tissues of the body such as lymph nodes, tonsils, adenoids, and the spleen. Lymphomas are separated into Hodgkin's and Non-Hodgkin's lymphomas. Hodgkin's disease primarily affects older adolescents. Any persistent, firm, nonpainful lump in the neck or armpits needs to be evaluated. Sarcomas are cancers that arise from connective tissue such as muscle or bone. Those that occur in bone, or osteosarcomas, typically occur during the major growth spurt of adolescence. The diagnosis may not be picked up early if symptoms of bone or joint pain are overlooked as "growing pains." Unexplained limping can also be a symptom. Neuroblastomas occur more frequently in infants and young children. Most are located in their adrenal gland. This tumor affects the sympathetic nervous system, a division of the autonomic nervous system that controls our involuntary bodily functions such as the goose bumps and rapid heartbeat that occur with fear. Look at your child's stomach when you are changing diapers or giving a bath. If you see a mass in the abdominal area, point it out for your doctor to examine. Finding an abdominal mass may also be a sign of the most common kidney tumor in children, a Wilm's tumor. This cancer is thought to arise from fetal kidney cells that fail to mature properly.

There are many nonspecific symptoms of childhood cancer. Some of these include unexplained weakness, constant nausea, lassitude, weight loss, and shortness of breath. Unexplained recurrent fevers or frequent bouts of infection should also make you suspicious. More specific symptoms of cancer may be things such as a persistent draining ear, a white dot in the eye, or any sudden change in vision. If a minor injury results in major bruising or extensive bruising just appears on your child's legs, take your child to the doctor for an evaluation. Any persistent lump or lumps in the neck, under the arm or in the abdominal area also need evaluation. Don't ignore swelling or pain in bones or joints. All these can be signs of cancer. In other words, pay close attention to all parts of your child's physical appearance and be aware of changes. Persistent and/or unusual changes may be a sign of cancer. Childhood cancer is relatively rare so your regular doctor may not put cancer on her differential diagnosis list on your first visit. You want cancer diagnosed as early as possible. Tell your doctor, out of earshot of your child, that you are worried about cancer. Don't wait for a subsequent visit.

In most cases the cause of the cancer is never found but, along with an inherited predisposition, the environment plays a big role in cancer development. Try to keep your children away from known toxic substances. The most well-known and common carcinogenic environmental toxin is smoke from tobacco products. Regular second-hand smoke inhalation has been associated with many kinds of cancer. Your child's environment should be smoke-free even if that means you or grandpa has to go outside to smoke. When that isn't possible, you may want to consider buying a good indoor air cleaner. To obtain more information about indoor air quality and health, go to the Internet and visit http://www.aerias.org or the main Air Quality Sciences, Inc., Web site at http://www.aqs.com.

Pay attention to labels on all insecticides and household chemical products that you buy and use them only as instructed. Store these products out of reach of children. When protective clothing isn't enough, make sure you use age-appropriate products on your child. Certain bug repellants have been specially formulated for use on children. These formulations contain lower amounts of chemicals such as the repellant DEET. Stronger formulations could be hazardous to your child. Make sure you apply repellants to areas of the skin or clothing that a small child can't lick or place in his mouth. Promptly and thoroughly wash the product off when it is no longer needed. Wipes and lotions are easier to use and prevent the possibility of inhalation of the aerosol.

Before swimming with young family members in local rivers, lakes, or streams, find out if companies and sanitation facilities dump waste materials in them. You may want to choose another water recreational area depending on what you discover. For example, microbial contamination of the Chattahoochee River in the metropolitan Atlanta area is being studied. As the result of treated wastewater dumping and untreated urban run off from leaking and overburdened sewers, microbial contamination has exceeded both Georgia and U.S. standards for recreation and fishing. The National Park Service has a Web site (http://ga.water.usgs.gov/projects/chatm) which posts the contamination studies and gives results. Look for similar Web sites covering parks and recreation facilities in your area before you let your child jump in and accidentally swallow water.

## Homicide

There are other health threats to children in addition to disease. Homicide ranks in the top five causes of death of children and young adults up to age twenty-five.[4] It is the most common cause of death for young black males in America. Whereas homicide of the elderly is usually committed by an unknown assailant, a family member is often the killer among homicide deaths of children younger than ten years old. Older children and adults are more apt to be killed by an acquaintance.

Frequent physical fighting during adolescence is the most important risk factor for homicide death in young males. Parents should practice and teach their children ways to settle conflicts other than through arguments and fist fights. Belonging to a gang also increases the risk of violent death, as gang members are more likely to own handguns. Parents should encourage social and afterschool activities such as sports, scouts, or youth groups that emphasize morals as an alternative to gang membership.

Substance abuse also contributes to homicide risk. The abused substance itself can induce violent behavior. Moreover, violence is often associated obtaining the necessary money to buy the abused substance. Many abusers resort to stealing, robbery, and other high-risk activities to support their habit. Lastly, since many abused substances are illegal, a high rate of violence is associated with the actual buying of these substances. To get their drugs, abusers may go to areas considered unsafe and associate with less than reputable individuals.

Be alert to changes in daily behavior and school or work performance as they may signal drug use. Use of alcohol and drugs can impair judgment, so an increase in accidents can also be a signal of drug and/or alcohol use. Because many drugs are inhaled or snorted, frequent coughing or sniffling without reason is common. If you notice any of these changes and suspect drug use, attempt to communicate with your child. If that proves to be unsatisfactory and you are still concerned and unsure, your doctor can run urine and blood tests that will detect the presence of commonly abused drugs. Many abused drugs are metabolized within forty-eight hours, so your child will need testing as soon as possible after you notice any unusual behavior. Your child may get very angry with you and may not want to submit to testing. As the parent, you will have to convince the child to give the urine specimen or to submit to having blood drawn. If your child is abusing drugs, you want them to get professional help as soon as possible. It is far better for your child to cry now than for you to cry later. Likewise, if you know a young adult exhibiting this kind of behavior, encourage him or her to get professional help.

# YOUNG ADULTS (YOU CAN AVOID SUICIDE, ACCIDENTS, AND HIV)

## Suicide

Suicide is a multifaceted condition. More medical attention needs to be paid to it because it ranks in the top five causes of death from adolescence up to middle age.[5] Ironically, spring, the time of rebirth, is the most popular season for suicide. Females attempt suicide more frequently than males, but males, especially white ones, are more successful and actually kill themselves more often. Males are more likely than females to use a violent method, which probably contributes to their higher success rate. Preadolescents are inclined to jump from heights and most suicides of young people occur within the home. Moreover, the presence of firearms in the home increases the chances of a suicide occurring since a method is readily available.

Feelings of hopelessness and worthlessness and a preoccupation with death or dying are common among those who commit suicide. Poor impulse control, a tendency toward antisocial behavior, and excessive risk taking are also typical behaviors. Be alert for these symptoms in yourself, your children, and in people you care about. If you have entertained thoughts of suicide and have figured out how to do it, or know someone who has a plan, it is urgent to seek help immediately. Many formulated plans for suicide are acted on because of the poor impulse control. Consequently, once a plan is made, it is imperative to get medical help immediately. Your primary care physician can help you or you may choose to see a psychiatrist. For help on the Web go to http://www.mentalhealth.org/suicideprevention.

Not surprisingly, substance abuse and mental disorders are also associated with suicide. Was the suicide in reality an accidental overdose? Perhaps the driving force behind the substance abuse was an attempt to self-treat an underlying mental disorder. In any event, depression and other mood disorders are diseases and should be treated. Individuals with mood disorders have a chemical imbalance in their brain just as diabetics have a shortage of insulin. Medicines such as the antidepressant Prozac can supply these chemicals and help restore life's balance. Typically side effects are minimal. If you hate to take pills, be aware that newer formulations exist with once-a-week dosing schedules. Hopefully, as medical knowledge increases about the chemical make-up of the brain, the social stigma associated with mental illness will disappear and more people will get medical help and not end up victims of suicide.

## Accidents

Accidents are the leading cause of death for everyone younger than twenty-five and rank in the top five causes of death until age sixty-five. Interestingly enough, most people don't talk to their doctor about accident prevention. Not surprisingly, motor vehicle injuries account for a large number of these deaths. Fasten your seat belt before you start your car. Teach your children to do the same. All fifty States, the District of Columbia, and Puerto Rico have adopted child seat belt laws because this is so important in saving lives. The rear middle seat is the best spot in the car to locate a child safety seat. Many public health departments run clinics where you can get your child seat inspected and learn how to install and use it properly. Call your local public health department or visit the National Highway Traffic Safety Administration Web site (http://www.nhtsa.dot.gov) to find the clinic nearest you. The Web site also has many pictures showing proper seat installation and a guide to the available types of child safety seats. Make sure you are wearing your own seat belt properly. Proper placement of your car seatbelt over your pelvic bones is important to protect your liver and your intestines in the event of a crash. If your seat belt is higher up, the belt can do severe damage to these internal organs without even breaking your skin. Your pelvic bones are strong and are likely to withstand the force of the impact but your liver and intestines can be severely damaged by sudden compression. You can bet supermodel Nikki Taylor is very careful about her seatbelt since recovering from the extensive liver damage she received as the result of an improperly positioned seat-belt when the car she was riding in crashed into a telephone pole.

When there is a new driver in the family, limit driving at night and don't allow unrelated passengers during the first 500 miles after licensure. New solo drivers don't need any distractions during this known accident-prone period. Many states are adopting graduated driving privileges for teenage drivers because these methods have been shown to lower the motor vehicle accident rate in this group. Even if your state hasn't adopted these policies, it is a good idea for you to at least limit the number of passengers. This is especially true in big cities with multiple lanes of fast moving cars where the slightest distraction can prove fatal.

Practice other preventive safety measures since falls, poisonings, fires and burns, and firearm injuries also cause significant loss of life. Simple things you can do that may save your life or that of a loved one include these:

▼ Don't drink and drive—many motor vehicle accidents involve alcohol consumption.
▼ Don't drink and participate in water related activities—many drownings and boating injuries involve alcohol consumption.
▼ Use motorcycle and bicycle helmets—the helmet may prevent a serious head injury.
▼ Properly install and maintain a smoke detector—many residential fire deaths could have been prevented by a working smoke detector.
▼ Safely store matches and lighters—children playing with these account for many residential fires.
▼ If you must smoke, don't do it in bed—bedding easily ignites, burns, and kills.
▼ Set hot water temperatures to 120–130 degrees Fahrenheit—prevent accidental scalding and more serious burns.
▼ If you own guns, keep them unloaded and stored in locked cabinets separate from the ammunition—many firearm deaths and injuries are unintentional.
▼ Safely store medicines and household products—prevent an accidental poisoning.
▼ Correct home environmental hazards that may cause falls—pay attention to loose rugs, unexpected objects, and inadequate lighting.

▼ Install window and stairway guards—keep someone from falling out a window or down stairs.

▼ Avoid placing furniture near unguarded windows and balconies—children may climb on the furniture and fall through.

## HIV

HIV, human immunodeficiency virus, is a major cause of death for men and women over age twenty-five and is rapidly becoming more common in younger age groups.[6] HIV infection affects both sexes, all races, and all economic groups but is more common in homosexual and bisexual males and in hypodermic drug users of either sex or any sexual orientation. Although treatment with newer medications is prolonging life, no cure currently exists. Researchers are trying to develop an effective vaccine to prevent the disease, but the task is daunting because of the complex nature of both the virus and our immune system. It is hoped a vaccine will become available within the next decade.

The most severe manifestations of a spectrum of illnesses caused by the virus are known as acquired immunodeficiency syndrome or AIDS. Infection with HIV eventually causes an individual to lose the protection of the body's immune system. As a result, the body can't ward off infections and cancers. Infected individuals develop unusual and rare infections and tumors that are very difficult to treat and often result in death. When a person is first infected with the virus, he is HIV-positive. AIDS begins when he or she starts exhibiting immune system failure by getting ill. The distinction is the severity of the compromise of the infected individual's immune system.

HIV is transmitted by *blood, semen,* or *vaginal fluid* from the infected individual coming in contact with someone else's *mucous membranes* or an *open cut.* Sexual intercourse is the most common means for the infected fluid to reach mucous membranes or an open wound. Transmission can occur through vaginal, anal, or oral sex. Although it is primarily sexually transmitted, you can also contract HIV by other means. You can be inoculated with the disease from a contaminated needle or syringe. Addicts and abusers who use needles to take drugs intravenously are at high risk for this type of transmission. In rare instances, healthcare workers have contracted the disease from a needle stick injury. (In other words, they were accidentally poked by a contaminated needle.) Having a blood transfusion was once a way to contract the disease but blood banks have been screening donors for HIV since 1985, so that is no longer likely. Unfortunately, pregnant women with HIV can infect their baby while it is in the womb, during childbirth, and through breastfeeding. Consequently, there is an increasing number of babies with the disease.

Transmission can also occur through open mouth or "French" kissing. The Centers for Disease Control (CDC) recommends avoiding "French" kissing with an infected individual. During this kind of kissing there is the potential for blood contact with the mucous membrane of the mouth because of bleeding gum disease and oral sores. There is no need to fear closed mouth or "social" kissing, as only the lips and cheeks are involved. Some people fear other means of transmission but no scientific evidence has been found to date to support those fears. Touching or other contact with saliva, sweat, or tears has not been shown to result in transmission of the virus. You do not need to worry about your waitress or waiter at a restaurant. Relax and enjoy your dinner.

As you increase your number of sexual partners, you increase your chances of contracting HIV. Although a latex or polyurethane condom, when used consistently and properly, does offer reasonable protection, having "safe sex" will not protect you completely from HIV. Abstinence is the only sure-fire protection. Even if the condom doesn't break, you are not completely protected, since transmission may occur during foreplay. The lubricating fluid released with arousal, prior to donning a condom, can be a source of infection. In addition, uncovered areas can come in contact with infected fluids anytime during the sex act. Natural membrane condoms, or "skins," do not offer any protection at all against HIV. Natural condoms have small pores that allow the virus to pass through, although they are too small for the passage of sperm and so prevent fertilization. The key is to *always use protection.* It is better to practice "safe sex" than be sorry the next morning. The need to use a condom outside of mutually monogamous relationships can't be overemphasized. Even if you are not concerned about a pregnancy because of a sterilization procedure or menopause, use a condom to protect yourself against HIV and other sexually transmitted infections. Remember, HIV and sexually transmitted diseases don't discriminate among ages. When you sleep with a person, you are sleeping with everyone else that he or she has slept with in terms of exposure to disease.

It can take up to six months after exposure to the virus for medical testing to detect the presence of HIV infection. As a result, a single HIV test is meaningless unless it is positive. If you think you may have been exposed, you need two negative tests spaced six months apart to be sure you have not contracted the virus. During the six-month period between tests, you need to abstain from all sexual contact and illicit drug use or you have to start the testing all over again. Many people have an AIDS test prior to entering a new sexual relationship. To truly ascertain your status and that of your desired new partner, you both need to abstain for six months and be retested prior to engaging in relations. To be really safe, in addition to HIV testing, you and your partner should be tested for other sexually transmitted infections such as gonorrhea, chlamydia, herpes, and syphilis. Infection with any other sexually transmitted disease enhances the transmission of HIV. In other words, if you have contracted another sexually transmitted infection and you have sex with an individual infected with HIV, your chances of catching HIV from him or her is increased.

Like other sexually transmitted infections, many people aren't aware initially that they have contracted HIV. If you develop any symptoms at all, they will mimic those of flu or mononucleosis. The symptoms may take days to weeks after exposure to occur, not the next morning, so it can be hard to trace them back to a specific lapse in judgment. Symptoms you may experience include fever, headache, malaise, nausea, sore throat, and joint and muscle aches. In addition, you may get a rash and/or ulcers on the mucous membranes of your mouth, your penis, or in and around your vagina. If you are at risk and you develop any unexplained febrile illness, request an HIV test. It may take from three weeks up to six months after these initial symptoms for seroconversion to occur, in other words, for the virus test to turn positive.

Many people are not diagnosed with HIV until after they start having problems with their health, such as frequent infections. If you are getting sick more often than usual, develop an unusual type of pneumonia or other rare infection and could possibly have been exposed, discuss the possibility of HIV with your doctor. Unless you mention current or past high-risk behavior, your doctor may not suspect the real culprit of your illness until much later in the course of the disease. Great strides have been made in the treatment of HIV that lengthens the time before full-blown AIDS develops. Treatment during the early phase of HIV infection can result in a slower progression of the disease process by preventing damage to the immune system and averting opportunistic infections. Thus it is to your advantage to be candid with your doctor and get diagnosed early in the course of the disease. Once you have seroconverted, careful medical monitoring will help you stay healthy as long as possible. If you know or suspect you have been exposed, have had a flu-like illness, and your initial test is negative, you may want to get retested every three to four weeks until you seroconvert or the six months is up.

## MIDDLE AGE (NEW CHALLENGES)

Having avoided birth defects, childhood cancer, accidents, homicides, suicides, and HIV, you now face the challenge of middle age. Besides distinguishing gray or thinning hair, you are subject to adult cancer, diabetes, atherosclerotic heart disease, and cerebrovascular accidents. For both sexes, heart disease is the number one killer, followed by cancer. The most common adult cancers are lung, colon and rectal, breast, and prostate.[7] Although only men get prostate cancer, both men and women can develop breast cancer, but it is far more common in women.

Certain factors statistically increase your chance of getting a particular type of cancer. These are called risk factors. However just because you have one, or two, or even all the risk factors for a cancer does not mean you will get that cancer. Doctors use risk factors to select individuals who are most likely to benefit from an early screening test or intervention. As mentioned earlier, testing can cause complications, so doctors want to make sure the benefit of a test out weighs any possible bad outcome caused by the testing procedure itself. Being aware of diseases that you have a greater than average chance of contracting empowers you to take charge of your health. By taking action you may be able to reduce your risk. For example, stopping smoking will lower your risk for many diseases including many cancers.

Being aware of your cancer likelihood can help you develop the personal self-awareness needed to recognize symptoms that may lead to an earlier diagnosis and a better prognosis. Diagnosed early, before spread or metastasis to other parts of the body has occurred, many cancers can be cured or controlled until you die of something else. You need to pay attention to your natural body rhythms so that you will be aware of small changes that can signal early disease. For example, how frequently do you have bowel movements and what shape and color are your stools? What is your normal energy level? How much sleep do you need to feel rested? Do you have new spots, bruises, or sores on your skin? Take the time to think about your daily body functions and seriously look at your body so that you have a good baseline in your mind for comparison.

Typically cancer does not cause pain in its early stage. Do not ignore mild symptoms because they're not painful. Symptoms that may signal early cancer and should be evaluated by your doctor include the following:

▼ A lump or thickening in the breast, testicles, or other body part
▼ A change in a mole or wart, or a new skin spot
▼ Any sore that will not heal
▼ A persistent cough or hoarseness
▼ A change in bowel or bladder habits
▼ Chronic indigestion or difficulty swallowing
▼ Any unexplained weight change
▼ Any unusual bleeding or discharge
▼ Persistent fatigue

Granted, the "c" word is probably the most frightening medical condition to deal with. However, when your doctor tells you that you have cancer, don't view it as a death sentence and panic. Your first reaction may well be "cut it out, now," but it is important to understand your treatment options. Don't rush into surgery. Take time to gain a full understanding of your cancer and the available treatment options. In most cases, delaying a few days won't affect your outcome but will empower you, with the help of your doctor, to select a treatment plan based on knowledge rather than fear.

## Lung Cancer

Lung cancer is the leading cause of cancer death in the United States for both men and women. It is a very difficult cancer to cure and has one of the worst prognoses of all cancers. Most people do not live five years after being diagnosed with lung cancer. The cancer spreads to nearby tissues, the liver, the brain, and to bone. Lung cancer is divided into two types, small cell cancer and non-small cell cancer, based on the appearance of the cancer cells when viewed underneath a microscope. Non-small cell cancer is more common and grows more slowly while small cell is a more aggressive and faster growing. There currently is no proven effective *screening* method for lung cancer although much research is being done in this area. Even if you are a smoker, no recognized medical group recommends having routine chest X-ray or sputum cytology testing to check for lung cancer *unless you have symptoms.* Abnormal growths in the lungs can be visualized by chest X-rays and the sputum cytology test looks at mucous you have coughed up under the microscope to see if cancerous cells are present. Both these tests are considered diagnostic tests, not screening tests, and thus are frequently used to make the diagnosis of lung cancer in symptomatic individuals. Until an effective screening test is found, it is up to you to pay attention to your body and report any unexplained changes to your doctor.

Tobacco use is associated with the majority of all lung cancers. In spite of this, people continue to smoke. Your best protection against lung cancer is to never use tobacco products and to avoid being with people when they smoke. Second-hand smoke has been shown to cause lung damage too, making the exposed nonsmokers more susceptible to lung cancer. Incidentally, although not a tobacco product, the smoke from marijuana, either inhaled or second-hand, also causes lung damage. If you smoke, your doctor has various methods to help you stop smoking. Talk to him about starting a smoking cessation program now. It is never too late to stop. Even if you develop lung cancer you should stop smoking because your outcome will be better. Another antismoking consideration is your appearance. Smokers develop facial wrinkles earlier than nonsmokers and face-lifts aren't covered by health plans. Smokers' teeth typically yellow more too, due to nicotine staining. As you can see, smoking is expensive to much more than your pocketbook.

Radon exposure is another known risk factor for lung cancer. Radon is a radioactive gas that occurs naturally in soil and rocks. It is invisible, odorless, and tasteless. If you live in an area known to contain radon, you may want to buy a kit to test for radon levels in your home, especially if your house has a basement or other rooms in the soil. Lack of good ventilation in the home due to closed or inadequate windows and outside vents can cause radon levels to build up to harmful levels in areas where radon is present. The test kits are inexpensive, readily available at hardware stores, and easy to use. To lower your risk of lung cancer you may just need to periodically open your windows. For more serious radon levels, inexpensive methods are available to decrease the amount of radon entering your home. You can get more information about radon control from the National Radon Information line at 800-SOS-Radon (800-767-7236) or from the National Safety Council at 800-557-2366. Online visit the Environmental Protection Agency's site about radon at http://www.epa.gov/iaq/radon.

Exposure to asbestos, a naturally occurring mineral whose crystalline shape is made up of long fibers, is known to cause lung cancer. Exposure at any level is felt to be a health hazard. The fibers can break with handling and send particles floating in the air that cause lung damage if inhaled. However, it is considered safe to use asbestos in products when it is properly bonded to another material to prevent the escape of fibers. Because it is heat resistant and a good insulator, asbestos has many industrial uses and was widely used in the construction of public buildings. The U.S. government stopped the production of most asbestos products in the 1970s because of health concerns and replaced or repaired materials in public buildings thought to pose a hazard. However, products that still use asbestos are readily available. These are primarily building materials used for heat and acoustic insulation, fireproofing, roofing, and flooring. Asbestos is also still used in friction products such as motor vehicle brakes and clutches. Industries producing such items provide protective clothing and recommend safe work practices for their employees. If you work for one of these industries, it is imperative you follow all safety procedures all of the time.

You may have asbestos-containing products in your home, especially if it was built prior to 1980. As long as the building material is in good repair, you probably do not have a hazard and should leave it alone. The greatest danger for exposure occurs with renovation work and demolition. If you are planning a home improvement project that could involve handling asbestos, you need to take proper precautions. Similarly, if you work on your own car and need clutch or brake repairs, be cautious. Manufacturers can tell you if their product contains asbestos and asbestos testing is available. To find an Environmental Protection Agency (EPA)-approved lab near you call 301-975-4016. The EPA has a very informative Web site that details safe sample collection, lists products containing asbestos, and provides related asbestos information at http://www.epa.gov/opptintr/asbestos/help.htm.

Another important risk factor for developing lung cancer is a history of previous lung disease that has left scarring in the lungs. The infectious disease tuberculosis is an example. Recurrent episodes of pneumonia can also scar your lungs. When lung-related symptoms take you to the doctor, you need to make sure to mention your past history of lung infections as this will alert her to put lung cancer higher up on the differential diagnosis list. Remember the goal is to make a diagnosis before the cancer has started to spread throughout the body.

Unexplained weight loss, loss of appetite, and fatigue can be early symptoms of any cancer, including lung. Symptoms of more advanced lung cancer may include chest pain, shortness of breath, wheezing, hoarseness, difficulty swallowing, and swelling of the face and arms. These symptoms develop as a result of the spread of the cancer throughout the chest cavity. Any cough that does not go away needs to be evaluated, even if you aren't a smoker. Nonsmokers get lung cancer, too. Always see your doctor if you cough up blood or blood-tinged phlegm. In addition, frequent bouts of bronchitis, pneumonia, or fever should make you think about the possibility of lung cancer.

## Colorectal Cancer

Colon or rectal cancer, also called colorectal cancer, affects both sexes and usually occurs after age fifty. The highest incidence is among African Americans. Colorectal cancer is the second most common cancer in the United States and, next to lung cancer, is responsible for the most cancer deaths. It is more likely to be located in the colon of women and in the rectum of men. The colon and rectum together make up what is known as the large intestine. The colon is the first six feet and the remaining eight to ten inches of intestine that connects to the anal opening is the rectum. (See figure 2, p. 38) The large intestine helps in the digestive process and in the formation, storing, and passage of stool. Thanks to the efforts of television celebrities such as Katie Couric, public awareness of this kind of cancer has increased. It is hoped that the empowered healthcare consumer will follow her lead and obtain appropriate screening. Early screening and diagnosis have been proven to lower the death rate from this cancer but many people still shy away from being screened. During screening, your modesty is protected by the use of drapes so don't let fear of exposure and embarrassment keep you from being diagnosed early.

Besides being over fifty, factors believed to increase your risk of getting colorectal cancer include having a first degree relative (parent, sibling, or child) with the disease, or if you have polyps, smoke, use alcohol, have a past medical history of other colon diseases, a personal history of other cancer, and a diet high in saturated fats. It is known that certain polyps, growths on the inner wall of the large intestine, can turn cancerous over a period of years. Polyps are relatively common in people over age fifty, but precancerous polyps are usually larger in size. Removal of these polyps is recommended to prevent later development of colon cancer. There are also certain inherited diseases involving the intestinal tract that contribute to the risk of colon cancer, so report any family history of bowel disease to your doctor. The majority of older individuals who develop colorectal cancer weren't at increased risk prior to their diagnosis. So don't think you can't get colon cancer because you don't have any of these risk factors. If you are fifty or older, you need to start regular screening for this disease.

The United States Preventive Services Task Force (USPSTF) currently recommends screening for colorectal cancer for all persons aged fifty and older. Annual fecal occult blood testing or periodic sigmoidoscopy or both can be used to accomplish the screening. The USPSTF felt there was insufficient scientific evidence at this point to recommend for or against using colonoscopy or a barium enema to screen *average risk* individuals. Their recommendations are continually being updated and the use of colonoscopy is being studied.

Fecal occult blood testing is easy to accomplish. The name describes the test. A small sample of stool or fecal matter is tested for blood not visible to the naked eye. If blood is found the test is considered positive and further testing to find the source of the blood is warranted. The doctor needs to find out if the blood is coming from a cancer or from something nonmalignant. The test examines stool so, for accuracy, dietary modifications need to have been followed for three to seven days to help prevent a false positive test. Substances that are known to irritate the bowel and could cause minute bleeding should be avoided. These include such things as aspirin, ibuprofen, and vitamin C. Eating foods rich in iron, such as red meat, can also cause a false positive test. Don't have the test if you are suffering from hemorrhoids, menstruating, have a urinary tract infection, or gingivitis, as these conditions are associated with bleeding and could cause a false positive test. Your doctor should give you a list of foods and medications to avoid when he gives you the stool collection cards.

Sigmoidoscopy involves inserting a lighted tube into the rectum and passing it up a part of the colon, the sigmoid colon, looking for any polyps or cancer. In sigmoidoscopy only the lower part of the colon can be examined, whereas colonoscopy, which also involves inserting a lighted tube up the rectum, can go much farther and look at the whole colon. This latter procedure has the advantage of allowing for biopsy of suspicious areas and removal of polyps during the examination. A barium enema is a series of X-rays of the large intestine after an enema of the contrast material, barium, has been given. The barium outlines the walls of the intestine, making it possible to see abnormalities on the X-ray. Unlike the fecal occult screening, the other screening tests require removing fecal material from the large intestine by means of oral laxatives and self-administered enemas prior to testing. Some patients find this cleansing of the bowel and the examination procedure uncomfortable. Your doctor can give you sedation for the testing if you are worried about the discomfort.

Make sure your doctor explains the risks associated with the various tests so you can decide together the best method of screening you for colorectal cancer. On the horizon is a new screening test that examines a single stool specimen for DNA mutations associated with colorectal cancer. This test holds great promise as it is noninvasive and specific for colon cancer. Hopefully, it will become available soon and add to your choices for screening.

Symptoms of colorectal cancer are related to bowel function except for the weight loss and constant tiredness that can come with any cancer. Imagine how having a growing mass in your large bowel would interfere with digestion and waste disposal. Clearly it would change your bowel habits. You may have general abdominal discomfort or frequent gas pains or cramps. You may feel an extra fullness or bloating. You may experience diarrhea, constipation, or a feeling of incomplete emptying. Your stools may become narrower than usual due to crowding from the mass. The mass could bleed or cause irritation resulting in bleeding. Thus blood might be seen in your stool. Blood color depends on the location of the bleeding in the colon. The blood would be bright red if the bleeding were lower down or dark red if from higher up. Don't just flush. Unless you start noticing the color, shape, and size of your stool, you could miss an early sign of a very common cancer.

## Breast Cancer

Breast cancer is the most commonly diagnosed cancer in women but lung cancer still causes more deaths. A pink ribbon worn on a collar or lapel has come to symbolize breast cancer, increasing the awareness of how many women are affected by this disease. It is estimated that every few minutes a woman is told she has breast cancer and every hour several women die from it. The disease affects white women more frequently than any other ethnic group. Men also get breast cancer, but, as previously noted, it is uncommon. October is National Breast Cancer Awareness month and, in 1993, President Bill Clinton proclaimed the third Friday of the month as National Mammography Day. On this day many radiologists provide discounted or free mammograms to promote and encourage breast cancer screening in women.

The breast is made up of fifteen to twenty lobes or well-defined groups within the breast. They are divided into many smaller lobules that become bulbs capable of producing milk. Thin tubes called ducts connect everything to the nipple. The breast also contains fatty tissue, blood vessels, and connections to lymph nodes. There is no muscle tissue in the breast but muscle does lie underneath the breasts and over the ribs. The most common breast cancer starts in the lining of the ducts and is called ductal cancer. Lobular cancer starts in the lobes of the breast. This kind of cancer is more likely to affect both breasts. Having big or little breasts does not increase or decrease your chances of getting breast cancer. No study has ever shown that breast size makes a difference.

As with other cancers, the usual suspects increase your risk of getting breast cancer. In other words, a family history of a first-degree relative with the disease, a personal history of cancer, and certain genetic alterations (BRCA1, BRCA2, and others) will increase your risk. In addition, a prior diagnosis of breast hyperplasia, a benign multiplying of normal cells found on biopsy of a breast mass, will increase your risk. Your age when your periods first began, your age at first giving birth, and your current age influence your risk. Menstruating before age twelve and/or first giving birth after age thirty are factors that increase the risk of cancer. However, the biggest risk most women face is just getting old. Breast cancer is relatively rare under age thirty-five; most breast cancer occurs in women over fifty. Other factors known to play a role in the development of breast cancer include taking hormones, a high fat diet, drinking alcohol daily, and lack of exercise. Having fibrocystic breast disease does not increase your risk of breast cancer but it can be harder to pick up a breast cancer in dense, lumpy breasts. To estimate your breast cancer current risk, you may want to use the tool developed by the National Cancer Institute found at http://bcra.nci.nih.gov/brc/q1htm.

If every woman in your family has developed breast cancer, you may have one of the genetic alterations associated with the disease. This is especially true if the women in your family have developed their breast cancer when they were still having menstrual periods. If this is the case, ask your doctor about undergoing genetic testing. If you do not have health insurance or your plan does not cover genetic testing, call your local chapter of the American Cancer Society to see if you qualify for an assistance program. If you can't locate them in the yellow pages, you can reach the national office at 800-ACS-2345 (800-227-2345) or you can visit them on the Web at http://www.cancer.org. If you have the gene alteration, ask your doctor for current information on research that is being done on drugs to prevent cancer. Tamoxifen is one drug that is currently being researched and most of the studies are promising.

You need to examine your breasts periodically so that you are aware of what normal is for you. Make breast examination part of your bathing routine. A woman's breasts change with her monthly periods, when on hormones or pregnant, and during the change of life. Use one of the readily available breast examination charts if you are uncertain of what to examine. The goal is to thoroughly examine your entire breast and under your armpit. Breast tissue can exist all the way under the arm. This is also where lymph nodes are located, so you don't want to miss this area. Be alert for any thickening or lump that persists. Many women get tender, lumpy breasts around their period but these changes go away after menstruation. Look at your breasts in the mirror. Be aware what the skin over your breasts looks like and the shape and size of each breast. It is normal to have one side slightly bigger than the other. Look at your nipples. Do they poke out or are they inverted? A cancer can change how a nipple protrudes. Check your bra to make sure there isn't any discharge. Nursing mothers may leak milk prior to a feeding but that is considered normal. If you notice anything different, see your doctor for further evaluation.

Early breast cancer typically is not painful. Some early symptoms that should make you insist upon an appointment for further evaluation include these:

▼ A change in the shape or size of a breast
▼ Ridges, pitting, inflammation, or dimpling of the skin over the breast
▼ A change in nipple appearance or a nipple being drawn back
▼ Nipple discharge, scaling, or tenderness
▼ A lump or thickening in the breast or underarm area

Routine screening for breast cancer every one to two years by mammography alone or in combination with an annual breast examination performed by a healthcare provider is recommended by the USPSTF for all women aged fifty to sixty-nine. Screening is not recommended for males. Other respected medical organizations recommend more frequent screening. However new evidence suggests that mammograms *may not* be as useful as once thought. This is still under investigation. In the meantime, ask your doctor to explain why he chooses to go with a particular group's screening recommendation. It is up to you, in partnership with your doctor, to evaluate your risk of breast cancer and decide what level of screening is best for you. If you are in a high-risk group, frequent screening may be appropriate.

A screening mammogram is the best tool doctors have to detect early breast cancer. A mammogram is a special X-ray that often can detect a breast mass before it can be felt. In addition, it can pick up calcifications that may be a sign of cancer. It is not a perfect test. A mammogram can be read as normal when a cancer is present even when a lump can be felt. A mammogram can be read as showing cancer when none is found on biopsy or lumpectomy. If you have a breast mass, don't depend on mammography alone. All breast lumps need *more* evaluation than just a mammogram.

Not all mammography centers are alike. Before you schedule an appointment, find out if the center meets the standard set in 1999 by the Mammography Quality Standards Act (MQSA). A center will be MQSA certified if they meet the standards developed by the federal government. Certification means the center you have selected performs a certain number of mammograms a year and has qualified technicians. You want to get the best mammogram possible. In addition, schedule your mammogram when you know your breasts won't be tender. To take the X-ray picture, your breast will have to be compressed by the X-ray machine. It is important to compress the breast during imaging to decrease the amount of thickness of the tissue the X-ray needs to pass through. This gives a clearer picture and makes abnormal areas more apparent to the radiologist. If you are tender, enough compression may not be applied to get the very best picture. If you are short and small breasted, asking the technician to lower the compression plates can make the procedure less awkward and less painful. Don't apply any deodorant or powder under your arms or on your chest area that day. Chemicals in these products can produce images on the X-ray film that may be confusing to interpret. You will have to undress from the waist up so it might be easier to wear pants or a skirt to your appointment rather than a dress. If you have had a mammogram in the past and are not returning to the same mammogram center, it is helpful to bring your old films with you. Just go to the center where they were taken before and ask for your films. This should be done beforehand. If this is not possible, bring the address of your previous center so your films can be sent for, if needed. Radiologists, doctors who interpret X-rays, like to compare the present mammogram with older ones to look for subtle changes.

Federal law mandates you be given your mammogram results.

The results will also go to your doctor. If you have not received your test results within two weeks, call the facility where your films were taken and ask for them. The law was passed to insure that women with positive or questionable mammograms are informed.

After a positive screening mammogram, you may need a diagnostic mammogram or special follow-up films to highlight a particular area of your breast. You may need an ultrasound study or a more invasive procedure to determine if you really have breast cancer. An ultrasound study uses high frequency sound waves to see if a breast lump is solid or fluid filled. A biopsy can be as simple as using a fine needle to withdraw fluid out of an area of the breast or it may involve having a lump surgically removed. If tissue is surgically removed, you need to have a sample of it taken for hormonal receptor testing. This testing helps determine if the hormones progesterone and estrogen, which naturally occur in a woman's body, are helping the cancer to grow. This test is important as it predicts the likelihood of responding to hormonal therapy should cancer be found. Depending upon your mammogram results, your doctor will discuss the best way to establish your diagnosis. Make sure you understand what is being suggested and why.

Today women with breast cancer have many treatment options. A mastectomy, removing the whole breast, may not be necessary. If you are told you have breast cancer, make sure you understand if the type you have is ductal, lobular, or something else. Find out the results of your hormone receptor tests and any other tests which were performed on the tumor, and be certain the doctor explains what these results mean in language you fully understand. Determine how your doctor plans on finding out if the cancer has already spread to other parts of your body. These questions need to be answered for you to have a good understanding of your prognosis, so you can make the best decision about the kind of treatment you want to undergo. You may want to consider a second opinion. Many health plans will cover the cost if it is requested. In fact, some insurance plans will require a second opinion before any surgical treatment is performed. It may take time to arrange for a second opinion, but brief delays of three to four weeks will likely not affect your outcome.

It will not make the cancer treatment you choose less effective, so take the time to find out all your options. Don't rush into a decision but carefully seek the best information available to you. Specialists who treat women for breast cancer include general surgeons, plastic surgeons, onocologists, and radiation onocologists. Special centers exist where only breast disease is treated. At these cancer centers, the specialists usually work as a team. Call the National Cancer Institute at 800-4-CANCER to find out about cancer centers and other cancer support programs in your area.

## Prostate Cancer

Prostate cancer awareness is just beginning to reach the public with the blue ribbon campaign. Since blue has traditionally been associated with baby boys, it is appropriate that a blue ribbon has been selected to represent the most common internal cancer affecting men. Prostate cancer kills more men than any other cancer except lung cancer. It is more common in African-American men and less common in Asian men and American Indians. The main risk factor for prostate cancer is age. Most men who get prostate cancer are usually well over age fifty. The average age at the time of diagnosis is about seventy. A family history of prostate cancer and a diet high in fat have also been associated with developing prostate cancer.

Prostate cancer is often an incidental autopsy finding in many men who die from other causes. The fact that many men with prostate cancer live normal lives and die of something else causes a medical dilemma. In some cases the cancer is very slow growing, stays within the prostate gland, and causes few problems. Cancer confined to the gland may exist for ten to fifteen years with no impact on life. In other cases the cancer grows rapidly, spreads, and ravages the body. Early in the disease process it is hard to know what the growth pattern of the cancer will be. Consequently, it is not known if early screening and detection of prostate cancer saves lives. To compound the issue, screening tests are not specific for just prostate cancer. Other nonmalignant diseases of the prostate gland can cause a positive screening test. The benefit of screening may not outweigh the risk of complications from the follow-up diagnostic testing that occurs with false positive results or the complications of treatment of cancers that end up being slow growing. Significant side effects that can change a man's life are possible as a result of the evaluation and treatment of this cancer. Men face the possibility of involuntary release of urine, known as incontinence, and the possibility of impotence, the inability to obtain an erection for sexual intercourse. Although medication such as Viagra can help with the impotence, as former senator Bob Dole has mentioned during television commercials, not everyone can safely take the drug. Products like Depends ease the embarrassment of urinary leakage but affected individuals still have to put up with the inconvenience of having to wear protection.

The prostate gland is a part of the male reproductive system (see figure 5). It is located in the pelvis and surrounds the urethra, the tube that carries urine from the bladder to the opening in the penis. In adults the prostate is about the size of a walnut. A doctor can determine the size and texture of the prostate gland by examining it through the rectal wall. To accomplish this, the doctor will ask you to bend over the exam room table while he inserts a lubricated, gloved finger into your rectum. During this digital rectal exam, the doctor is looking for enlargement, lumps, or induration that might be a sign of cancer or other prostate disease.

The cells of the prostate gland secrete and store a fluid that combines with sperm from the testicles to make semen. Semen is released from the penis during sexual climax. The prostate is divided into three zones: the peripheral, the central, and the transitional. Most cancer occurs in the peripheral zone farthest away from the urethra, so a man can have early prostate cancer without urinary symptoms. The prostate gland normally enlarges as the result of aging. This is known as benign prostatic hypertrophy, or BPH. This enlargement typically occurs in the transitional zone located near the urethra, causing symptoms of urethral irritation, such as frequent urination and awakening at night and having to go. However, prostate cancer can produce similar symptoms as those of the normal aging process, so you should see your doctor at the onset of symptoms. Don't brush your symptoms off as just part of getting old. You are not wasting

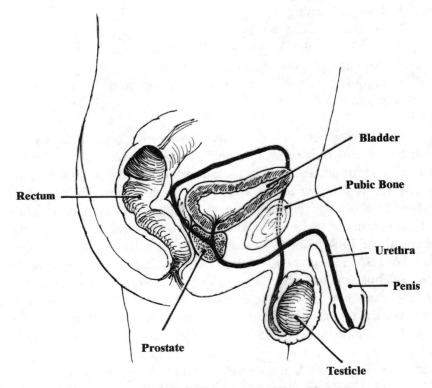

**Bladder**

**Pubic Bone**

Rectum

**Urethra**

**Penis**

Prostate

Testicle

# Figure 5. Male Reproductive System

illustration by Elizabeth Vance, adapted from Rx Humor (www.dochollywood.com)

your time going to the doctor, because even if cancer is not found, medication is available to treat the inconvenient and embarrassing symptoms associated with BPH.

Because of its location and function, symptoms that could indicate prostate cancer involve urination and sexual function. Prostate cancer, as it grows, impinges on the urethra and spreads locally to the bladder and other nearby tissue. It can spread through both the lymph and blood systems to distant locations such as the spine and bones. Common symptoms include the following:

▼ The need to urinate frequently, especially at night
▼ Difficulty initiating urination
▼ Weak or interrupted urine stream

▼  Pain or burning with urination
▼  Difficulty having an erection
▼  Painful erection
▼  Presence of blood in urine or semen
▼  Frequent pain or stiffness in the lower back, hips, or upper
    thigh area

The fluid secreted by the cells of the prostate gland contains a substance known as prostate specific antigen (PSA). The blood test that checks for prostate cancer measures levels of this substance. Normally levels are low in the blood and high in the prostate gland where PSA is made. However, anything that disrupts the architecture of the prostate gland such as a cancer or an infection causes greater amounts of PSA to be released into the circulation. A high blood level of PSA reflects the disruption of the cells, but does not give the cause. Thus, it is not a specific test for prostate cancer. Levels of PSA greater than 4 ng/ml may be suggestive of cancer. Methods are used to make the test more specific for cancer such as adjusting levels for age. In addition, specialized PSA tests are now becoming available. The free PSA test is a specialized test that looks at the amount of the differing forms of PSA in the blood. PSA circulates in the blood both freely and bound to a protein molecule. With cancer more of the PSA is in the bound form. Consequently a free PSA level of less than 25 percent of the total PSA level is suggestive of cancer.

Although the USPSTF does not recommend routine screening for prostate cancer, the American Cancer Society feels that all men over age fifty should be offered an annual PSA level and a digital rectal exam. In the case of prostate screening, the medical world has been unable to reach consensus because early detection of prostate cancer has not yet been proven to extend life. Consequently, at age fifty, in addition to blowing out birthday candles, it is time to discuss prostate cancer screening with your doctor and decide what is best for you.

Remember, if you are screened for prostate cancer and the results come back positive, you still may not have cancer but follow-up is necessary. However, if a nodule is felt on digital rectal exam, it will need to be biopsied. In addition, follow-up of some elevated PSA levels may also require a biopsy. One way to obtain a biopsy is through the rectum, using ultrasound to guide the needle. Discuss with your doctor the kind of biopsy that is planned, how long the procedure will take, and how soon you can expect the results.

If your subsequent diagnostic testing is positive for prostate cancer, you need to be involved in the decision about treatment. In addition to how advanced (stage) your cancer is and how aggressive (grade) your cancer is, your age and general health status will play a key factor in the decision making process. Many older men have other illnesses that pose a greater threat to their survival than the prostate cancer. In certain instances, where you have the more benign kind of cancer, the best thing may be to do nothing. Just waiting to see what happens can be the best treatment. The goal of treatment should be to maintain your quality of life while increasing your survival. As with any other cancer, you may want to get a second opinion. Don't rush into treatment without investigating your options. Following are crucial questions to discuss with your doctor:

▼ What are the expected benefits of the proposed treatment?
▼ What are the risks and side effects of the proposed treatment?
▼ What is the probability of your sex life being affected?
▼ What is the likelihood of having urinary problems as a result of treatment?
▼ What is the likelihood of having bowel problems as a result of treatment?
▼ Do you qualify for any new treatments under study?

## Heart Disease

Heart disease presents a much bigger risk to our lives than the cancer most of us fear. Perhaps this is because we have visions of a lingering death with cancer and a sudden and swift one from heart disease. More people die from heart disease than any other illness. This is true even when all kinds of cancer are combined. Symptoms of heart disease can be mild, even when extensive disease is present, because, although many blood vessels are involved, flow to the heart can still be maintained. As a result, screening electrocardiograms (EKGs) do not do a good job of predicting who will experience a heart attack. If blood flow to the coronary vessels is maintained during the test, the results are normal. The same is true when an EKG is done during exercise—a stress EKG. Stories abound of someone literally dropping dead from a massive heart attack after being told they had a normal EKG. A newer test, electron beam computed tomograghy (EBCT), can detect calcifications in the coronary arteries. Calcium is believed to be a marker for atherosclerosis and thus a predictor of heart disease. However, the absence of detectable coronary artery calcification, a negative test, does not completely rule out the presence of atherosclerosis and the possibility of heart disease. Likewise, the presence of calcification, a positive test, does not mean you will have a heart attack, only that you have a higher risk. Newer screening blood tests which indicate inflammation levels in the blood are currently being studied and may end up being good predictors for heart disease. In all likelihood no test will ever be a perfect predictor of the disease. However newer medications are able to bust clots and stop some heart attacks before permanent damage occurs. These medications must be administered quickly after heart attack symptoms develop, so *call 911 immediately when a heart attack is suspected!*

Heart disease is thought of as a man's disease. However, this is not true. Heart disease will also kill more women than all forms of cancer combined. Men start getting heart attacks at a younger age but, after menopause, women catch up. Being a male over forty-five years old or a female over fifty (or postmenopausal) increases your risk for heart disease. The symptoms of heart disease may not be as pronounced in women, so it is especially important for women to pay attention to what their body is telling them.

When blood flow to an area of the heart is impeded, chest pain may develop. If this occurs when you engage in activity, it is known as angina, and it is the most common warning symptom of heart disease. Unfortunately many people don't have this warning symptom, or chose to ignore it, and discover their heart disease only by having a heart attack. Completely blocked blood flow to a section of the heart causes that area to die, or to become infarcted. Hence the term "myocardial infarction" is used for a heart attack. Blockage can occur within the blood vessel itself by way of a deposit or plaque, or it can occur by pieces of a plaque located elsewhere breaking off and then lodging and clogging the vessel. The severity of any heart attack depends on the vessel or vessels affected. (See figure 4, "Anatomy of the Heart," p. 76.) If a large enough area of the heart is infarcted, death occurs rapidly.

Smoking is the most avoidable risk factor for cardiovascular disease. In addition to causing cancer, tobacco use increases your chances of a heart attack. Cigarette commercials never show someone grasping at their chest and falling over dead, but they should. If you smoke, ask your doctor about the nicotine-containing gum, patches, and inhalers available to help you avoid nicotine withdrawal symptoms when stopping smoking. If someone in your household smokes, make them go outside. Being around smokers and inhaling second-hand smoke also increases your risk of heart disease. Besides protecting your heart, you are doing others a favor by making it more difficult for them to indulge in a very dangerous habit.

High blood pressure is the silent killer. Many people are unaware that their blood pressure is high until they have a heart attack or stroke. Even people who know they have high blood pressure often ignore it or fail to take their medication because they don't feel bad. You don't have to see a doctor to find out your blood pressure. Reliable blood pressure machines are located at most drug stores. If you have a high reading on either number, make an appointment to see your doctor for an evaluation. Both numbers, the top, or systolic, and the lower, or diastolic, should be within the normal range. Blood pressure is considered normal in people over the age of eighteen if the systolic reading is 130 or less and the diastolic is 85 or less. This would be charted as a reading of 130/85. Optimal blood pressure is a reading of 120/80 or less. Black men are especially prone to high blood pressure so they may want to read the book *The Black Man's Guide to Good Health* written by Drs. James Reed and Neil Shulman.[8] Many people with hypertension don't take their medicine because of side effects. Talk to your doctor. Don't be embarrassed to discuss what the medicine is doing to your sex life. Many different medications and the medical device RESPeRATE are available to help control your pressure. Your doctor can switch medications so that both your pressure and the side effects are acceptable.

Cholesterol is a waxy fat that can form thick deposits, known as plaques, on blood vessel walls. Thus, a high total cholesterol level in the blood is associated with heart disease. The plaques make the vessel harder and restrict or obstruct blood flow through it, which can cause a heart attack. Your body produces some of your cholesterol in the liver and the rest comes from the animal products you eat. Fruits and vegetables do not contain cholesterol, although vegetable oils do contain fat. However, in cooking fresh vegetables, especially baked potatoes, many of us top them with cholesterol-containing butter for flavor.

Your blood has two kinds of cholesterol: high density (HDL) and low density (LDL). High density is the good kind of cholesterol because it protects from heart disease. It is thought that HDL helps carry cholesterol away from the vessels and back to the liver. Low density is the bad kind, or heart-attack–causing cholesterol, because it encourages plaque formations. As a result, you need to know your total cholesterol level and the amount of both good and bad cholesterol in your blood to determine your risk of heart disease. In addition, watch the fat content of your diet. Diets high in fat, especially saturated fats, are associated with higher cholesterol levels. Consider putting no-fat sour cream instead of butter on that baked potato.

Regular exercise and maintaining healthy body weight also helps stave off heart disease. Exercise benefits the heart in many ways. It has been shown to lower blood pressure, to increase HDL levels, and to decrease weight. Try to incorporate more activity in your daily routine. For example, take the stairs instead of an elevator and park in the back of the lot instead of circling for a close spot. Obesity is also a factor in developing diabetes. Diabetes, which affects your body's ability to control your blood sugar level, also increases your likelihood of having cardiovascular disease. Many diabetic patients are also overweight and don't exercise regularly so they get a triple whammy. Couch potatoes, beware. As you eat fast food filled with fat, your waistline gets bigger and you increase your chance for heart disease and diabetes. Think about your heart the next time you reach for the bowl of chips while clicking the TV remote control.

Of course, family history plays a factor in heart disease. This is particularly true if the men in your family had a heart attack prior to age fifty-five or the women were affected under age sixty-five. However, don't think you are safe just because no one in your family has had a heart attack or stroke. Remember you don't have to have a risk factor to get a disease and heart disease is the number one killer in the United States. Current research suggests a correlation between smoldering inflammation in the blood stream and heart attacks to explain the number of people who get heart disease without any known risk factors. This research also helps explain why taking a baby aspirin daily can help prevent a heart attack. In addition to thinning the blood and slowing clotting, aspirin blocks inflammation. You should discuss with your doctor whether or not you should start taking daily aspirin to help ward off heart disease.

You may experience angina as a warning signal prior to actually having a heart attack or you may get leg pain with walking, known as claudication. With claudication the blood flow to the legs is impeded but the flow to the heart is sufficient so leg pain, not chest pain, occurs. You may get chest pain with any activity requiring increased blood flow to the heart such as fast walking or being outside in the cold. Typically angina lasts briefly and clears with stopping the activity. The chest pain associated with a heart attack usually lasts longer. No chest pain should be ignored. It does not need to be severe. Any unpleasantness, discomfort, or heaviness in the chest area should be evaluated. This is particularly true of women, who tend to have more subtle symptoms. Words that heart attack victims use to describe their chest pain include "pressing," "squeezing," "strangling," "constricting," "burning," and "bursting." The pain will sometimes also move, or radiate, to the upper arms, neck, or jaw. Typically the pain starts in the chest and then radiates to the other areas but, instead of chest pain, you might just have an unexplained pain, heaviness, or discomfort in the upper arms, neck, or jaw.

Another warning sign of a heart attack or heart disease is shortness of breath. If you become uncomfortably aware of your breathing, you should consider your heart. It is normal to get short of breath with exercise, especially if you are out of shape. However, shortness of breath at normal activity levels or at rest should be taken seriously and evaluated by your doctor. Other symptoms that should not be ignored include persistent or unusual indigestion, heartburn, or nausea and unusual fatigue or breaking into a cold sweat for no reason. In other words, if you are dragging, your chest feels a little tight, and you break out into a cold sweat, think heart attack. *Call 911 and take an aspirin.* That television commercial is correct: Taking an aspirin will increase your chances of survival if you are having a heart attack.

## Stroke

Stroke and heart disease risks are intermingled. The factors causing one also cause the other. Instead of involving the blood supply to the heart, in strokes the flow to the brain is affected. In this sense, a stroke can be looked on as a "brain attack." The biggest difference is that strokes tend to occur later in life; most people experience strokes after age sixty-five. Slightly more men than women have strokes and the highest incidence occurs among blacks. Stroke survivors can place a tremendous burden on family members and caretakers because recovery is often incomplete.

A stroke occurs when blood flow to an area of the brain stops due to vessel breakage or vessel blockage. The surrounding brain cells die and the area of body control served by those cells is lost. The majority of strokes occur because a clot formed within the vessel or one came from elsewhere, such as the carotid artery in your neck, to block a vessel. This is known as an ischemic stroke. Less frequently, a stroke occurs when a vessel in the brain breaks and bleeds into the surrounding brain tissue. This is known as a hemorrhagic stroke. The end result, loss of brain and body function, is the same but the treatment is different. Your doctor will order tests to determine what kind of stroke has occurred.

Brain cells are very sensitive to oxygen deprivation. If blood does not flow to an area of the brain, the cells can't get oxygen or glucose and die. When complete blood flow is cut off to the brain, unconsciousness results within ten seconds. However, it is rare for all the blood supply to the brain to be cut off. With a stroke, usually an area of the brain loses only its main blood supply. Some flow is maintained because of collateral circulation. The longer an area of the brain remains only marginally supplied with blood, the less likely the affected brain tissue is to fully recover. Consequently, stroke treatment must be initiated within two to six hours of the onset of symptoms to have a chance at preventing irreversible brain damage. Brain cells do not grow back, so other areas of the brain have to be trained to compensate for the loss of function. This process is known as rehabilitation and takes many weeks. The severity of the stroke and the area of the brain affected determine how much and what body functions can be restored. The left side of the brain controls the right side of the body and vice versa. (Figure 6 depicts the areas of the brain.) In addition, each side of the brain controls various specialized perceptual tasks such as spatial orientation and language abilities. The cerebellum controls coordination and balance and the brain stem controls basic body support functions which we don't think about, such as breathing. Typically a stroke will involve only one side of the body, but those that involve the brain stem can affect both sides. Rehabilitation focuses on relearning skills necessary for daily living such as eating, toileting, dressing, physical movement, and provides other skills to deal with cognitive and language impairments.

Strokes may be preceded by a reversible interference of blood flow to the brain known as a transient ischemic attack or TIA. The blood supply to a part of the brain is briefly interrupted producing symptoms similar to a stroke. The attack comes on suddenly, without warning, and maximum intensity is almost immediate. The symptoms vary depending on the part of the brain affected. They usually last less than thirty minutes, but can continue up to twenty-four hours. Recovery is complete but a thorough medical examination is warranted in hopes of preventing a future stroke or heart attack. If the cause can be found, medical or surgical treatment may be indicated to prevent future attacks. If you experience *any transient loss of body or cognitive function, you should seek medical attention.* For example,

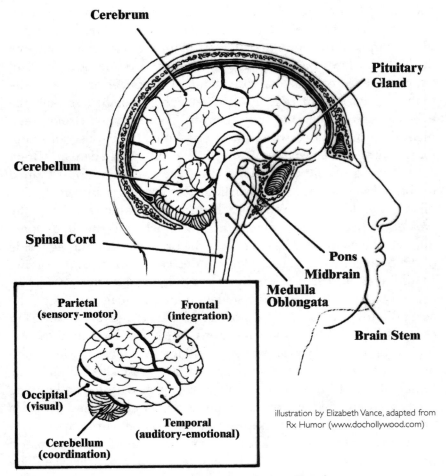

Figure 6. Areas of the Brain

if you experience slurred speech for a few minutes and you haven't been drinking, you may have had a TIA. Or perhaps you feel like a shade was temporarily drawn over your eye, or, momentarily, written words were incomprehensible. The loss of function correlates with the area of the brain that is not getting enough blood. When the flow is restored, the symptoms go away but the danger of a reoccurrence which will leave permanent damage is high.

The difference between a TIA and a stroke is really a matter of duration of symptoms. A stroke also comes on suddenly without provocation. However, by definition, the symptoms of a stroke last longer than twenty-four hours. The symptoms are most severe usually within an hour of onset. The pattern of symptom development can give your doctor diagnostic clues so it is helpful for a family member or friend to supply these details if you are incapacitated. As with a TIA, the area of the brain affected determines the symptoms. Symptoms suggestive of a stroke or TIA include the following:

▼ Any sudden weakness or loss of sensation to the arm, face, or leg
▼ Any sudden unexplained bout of confusion or lack of understanding
▼ Any sudden trouble with your vision
▼ Any sudden loss of coordination or balance or trouble walking
▼ Any sudden and severe headache with no known cause

Atrial fibrillation, a common heart rhythm abnormality in the elderly, increases your risk for a stroke. In this condition, the upper chambers of the heart don't beat correctly. The abnormal beating may cause a blood clot to form in the heart and be carried to the brain, triggering a stroke. Most affected elderly patients are treated with medications to help prevent this occurrence but treatment is not always successful. Another condition associated with an increased incidence of stroke is carotid artery stenosis. In this condition, atheroscleortic plaques form in the main vessels that carry blood to the head, the carotid arteries. The plaques can interfere with blood flow to the brain. With severe obstruction or after a TIA, surgery is sometimes suggested to remove the plaque formation in one or both of the carotid arteries in hopes of preventing a stroke.

Depending on the area of the brain affected, a stroke can be devastating. It can leave you paralyzed on one side of your body and unable to swallow. You may lose your ability to see normally out of an eye or to even process language and talk normally. You don't want to have a stroke. While some of the factors are uncontrollable, such as your family history, age, and gender, there are things you can do to help prevent a stroke. If you have high blood pressure, make sure it is controlled. Take your medication as prescribed and follow-up with your doctor as directed. Don't use tobacco products. If you currently smoke, stop. Blood pressure control and smoking cessation are the most effective interventions available for preventing strokes.

## Diabetes Mellitus

Diabetes Mellitus increases your risk of having a stroke or heart attack and is a leading cause of death in adults. In addition, it is the leading cause of adult blindness in the United States, is responsible for the majority of nontraumatic limb amputations, and is a major cause of kidney failure. Diabetes basically comes in two forms, although others exist. The most common form is known as Adult Onset diabetes, Type 2 diabetes, or Noninsulin Dependent diabetes (NIDDM). The other form is known as Juvenile Onset diabetes, Type 1 diabetes, or Insulin Dependent diabetes (IDDM). Insulin, a hormone produced in the pancreas, allows cells in our body to burn sugar for fuel. Both forms of diabetes result in high blood sugar levels because the body does not produce enough insulin or is resistant to the presence of insulin. As the name implies, people with IDDM need insulin shots for treatment but those with NIDDM can usually control their disease through oral medication and diet. Complications of the disease are divided into those affecting small blood vessels and those affecting large blood vessels. The small, or microvascular, complications are those that involve the retina of the eye, nerves, and the kidneys. Examples are blindness, loss of sensation to the feet, and kidney failure. The large, or macrovascular, complications are those associated with atherosclerosis such as heart attacks, strokes, and gangrene.

IDDM involves the destruction of the cells in the pancreas that make insulin. NIDDM is a problem of insulin resistance. The pancreas still makes insulin but the body cells ignore or become resistant to it so higher levels than normal are required. Family history is a factor in both forms of the disease but especially so with NIDDM. Usually young people get IDDM although it can occur at any age. People over forty are more likely to get NIDDM. Blacks, Hispanics, and Native Americans are at greatest risk for the disease. Women who temporarily have diabetes during pregnancy, known as gestational diabetes, are at a higher risk of developing permanent diabetes later in life.

Poor physical fitness is associated with insulin resistance and can lead to the onset of diabetes. In addition, smoking and obesity also increase the risk of developing diabetes. Clearly these are areas of personal control. You need to make healthy decisions about your life. Part of being an empowered healthcare consumer is making tough decisions and being proactive about your health. You can lower your risk of this major killer by not smoking, by participating in regular exercise, and by maintaining a healthy weight. You do not have to gain weight as you get older. Most age-related weight gain is attributed to decreased activity without a reduction in consumption. Weight control is not rocket science. The more you eat, the more you must move if you don't want to gain.

Symptoms of diabetes result from excessive sugar levels in the blood. In an attempt to lower your sugar levels, your kidneys put sugar into your urine. The sugar is like a sponge and carries fluid out of the body in the form of urine. Consequently you are always thirsty and urinate frequently. Your body can't effectively utilize the sugar as fuel so you are hungry and eat more than usual but still lose weight. Additionally you may experience blurred or other changes in your vision and become more susceptible to simple infections. However, a significant number of people with NIDDM have no symptoms. It is possible to have diabetes for many years and not be diagnosed until a complication arises. Consequently, if you are at risk for the disease by being overweight, over forty, and sedentary, ask your doctor to test you for diabetes. This is especially true if the disease runs in your family. There are currently no recommendations for or against routine screening for diabetes, although it is recommended for those at risk. Thus, it is up to you to request testing.

There are many ways to test for diabetes. Before a doctor makes a definitive diagnosis, you should have an abnormal test on more than one occasion. To get the most meaningful results, you should eat normally for three days and then fast overnight prior to the test. Typically an abnormal fasting blood sugar level is followed up with an oral glucose tolerance test. In this test you are given a drink containing glucose, a sugar, and your blood is drawn at set intervals to see how quickly your body metabolizes the sugar. Once the diagnosis of diabetes has been made, it is up to you to take control of the disease. You need to achieve good blood sugar control. Good blood sugar control has been shown to slow the onset of microvascular complications of the disease. Control is accomplished by taking medication as directed and following a diabetic diet. Sometimes insulin is needed, even in NIDDM, to get control. It is better for your long-term health to take insulin shots to get control than to be only partially controlled with oral medication. Other things that will help are a regular exercise program and weight loss if you are heavy. Exercise increases insulin sensitivity and weight loss lowers your insulin needs. Many people with NIDDM manage their disease without medication just by losing weight and watching what they eat. They make the effort and gain control of their health.

Because diabetes can affect all organs of your body, it is important that you schedule regular follow-up visits with your doctor. How often you need to been seen will depend on your level of blood sugar control. At least twice a year all diabetics should take a glycalated hemoglobin or HbA1c test. This test is a measure of your average blood sugar levels over the prior two to three months. In other words, even if your blood sugar level is okay on the day of your visit, your doctor will be able to tell if your sugar wasn't in control most of the time. In addition, during these check-ups, your doctor should closely examine your eyes, cardiovascular system, and feet in order to pick up early signs of diabetic complications.

## SENIOR CITIZENS (GOLDEN YEARS?)

For the elderly, Chronic Obstructive Pulmonary Disease (COPD), pneumonia, and influenza (flu) become leading causes of death.[9] Immunization can prevent some types of pneumonia and the flu but the only protection from COPD is not smoking. We lose some lung capacity as a normal part of aging and that, combined with underlying diseases such as heart disease, leaves us more susceptible to pneumonia and flu. Living in nursing homes and other assisted living facilities increases the exposure to organisms that cause lung infections. It is not surprising that the greatest number of pneumonia and flu deaths occur among people over age eighty-five. More men than women get pneumonia and blacks have a higher incidence than Caucasians. Having COPD also increases the risk of contracting pneumonia and flu.

## Pneumonia

Pneumonia produces an inflammation in the lung tissues and can be caused by a bacterial, viral, or chemical irritant. For example, if you vomit and aspirate some of the material into your lungs or inhale smoke in a fire you can get a severe chemical pneumonia. Symptoms vary with the causative agent, but most pneumonia is associated with fever and a productive cough. The mucous or sputum that is coughed up may be discolored, thick, or scanty. The color of the phlegm can suggest the infectious agent. For example, rust colored sputum is associated with bacterial pneumococcal pneumonia. Chest pain and fast breathing at rest are also symptoms of pneumonia, as is shortness of breath with normal activity.

On physical exam your doctor may hear abnormal sounds when he listens to your chest. If he suspects pneumonia, a chest X-ray should be ordered to confirm the diagnosis. Treatment will involve antibiotics for bacterial pneumonias along with supportive care such as oxygen.

Recently there has been an increase in reported cases of bacterial pneumonias that are resistant to treatment by antibiotics, even to the newer ones. Consequently, prevention through vaccination is more important than ever. Vaccination to prevent pneumonia is recommended for all people over sixty-five and those at risk for the disease. You are considered to be at risk if you suffer from a chronic debilitating disease such as COPD or live in a nursing home or an assisted living facility. The vaccine is typically given as a one time only shot but certain individuals may need a booster shot in five years.

## Influenza

Influenza A and B viruses cause the flu. The virus enters the body through the mouth, nose, or the eyes, and then invades the lining of the respiratory system. When a sick person coughs, the virus becomes airborne, spreading the disease to others. Susceptible individuals become sick one to four days after exposure. You can get the flu more than once since the viruses that cause the disease constantly change their appearance, fooling your body's protective immune system. Consequently, yearly immunization (getting a flu shot every year) is the best protection. Flu occurs most often in the winter months, so October and November are the best time to be immunized. The shot starts working within ten to fourteen days after being administered and is highly effective.

You may confuse symptoms of the flu with those of a bad cold. However, with the flu the onset is more rapid and severe. If you are feeling fine one moment and the next you feel like you have been hit by a truck, check and see if there has been a flu outbreak in your area. See table 3 for further differentiation between flu and colds.

New antiviral medications are available that can be used to treat the flu to lessen the severity and the length of the illness. To be effective, the medication needs to be started within forty-eight hours of the onset of symptoms. The medication can also prevent the occurrence of flu when taken within two days after exposure to the disease. If you think you have the flu, or have been exposed to flu, you need to see your doctor immediately to benefit from this treatment.

## Chronic Obstructive Pulmonary Disease

Chronic obstructive pulmonary disease (COPD) worsens with time, unlike pneumonia and flu where a complete recovery is possible. There is no cure for this disease. The hallmark is a progressive and permanent decline in lung function interspersed with periodic acute

| TABLE 3. FLU VERSUS COLD SYMPTOMS ||
| Flu Symptoms | Cold Symptoms |
| --- | --- |
| Sudden onset | Gradual onset |
| Fever over 101 | Absent or low grade fever |
| Headache | Headache usually not present |
| Muscle aches and pains | Mild muscle aches/pains, if any |
| Exhaustion | Mild fatigue, if any |
| Sneezing and congestion uncommon | Sneezing and congestion common |

attacks. The damage caused to the lungs is irreversible. Whites are affected more frequently than blacks and men more than women. However, the number of women suffering from this disease is increasing, a statistic attributed to the increased number of women who are now smoking. A small number of cases are associated with an inherited deficiency of the substance Alpha 1Antitrypsin, but most cases are caused by smoking and second-hand smoke inhalation.

COPD is characterized by airflow obstruction in the lungs caused by emphysema, chronic bronchitis, or a combination of both. The lung is made up of airways, or bronchial tubes, to bring the air in and air sacs, or alveoli, to transfer oxygen and carbon dioxide to and from the blood. Bronchitis causes inflammation of the lining of the large and small bronchial tubes. This leads to increased mucous production, plugging, and scarring of the airways. As the disease progresses, it becomes increasingly difficult to get air down to the air sacs. In emphysema the air sacs of the lung become less elastic, weaken, break, and trap air. Consequently oxygen is not effectively transferred to the blood and carbon dioxide is inadequately removed. In either case the body gets less oxygen. People suffering from COPD become short of breath with any activity that increases the amount of oxygen used by the body. COPD can become so severe that, even with supplemental oxygen, it can be difficult to bathe or get dressed because of shortness of breath.

The most common symptoms of COPD are chronic coughing and shortness of breath. The breathlessness increases with an acute flare-up. Increased cough and sputum production, wheezing, and fever also may signal an acute episode. If you have a chronic cough and get short of breath most days, you need to see your doctor. Don't just assume you are getting old and are just out of shape. If you smoke you probably ignore your morning "smoker's cough" and don't pay too much attention to the "bad colds" you periodically get during the year. However, you are likely experiencing early COPD. Make an appointment now to find out how much damage you have already done to your lung capacity. By having you breathe into a machine, your doctor can measure how deeply you are able to breathe and how fast you can move air in and out of your lungs. Perhaps if you learn how much of your lung function you have already lost, you will finally quit smoking.

Since there is no cure for COPD, the goal of treatment is to increase the quality of life while decreasing breathlessness. Multiple pills and inhalers may be prescribed that have varying methods of action. Staying as physically fit as possible is important since strong muscles perform more efficiently and use less oxygen. A new surgical procedure called lung volume reduction surgery may offer some hope of improving lung function in patients with severe disease. As you can see, with COPD, an ounce of prevention is worth a pound of cure.

## Alzheimer's Disease

Alzheimer's disease is perhaps even more heartbreaking than suffering from cancer or a stroke. Alzheimer's disease is an irreversible, progressive, degenerative disease of the brain that ultimately leads to dementia and death. It is the most common cause of permanent dementia in adults. Former president Ronald Reagan is perhaps the most prominent individual suffering from Alzheimer's disease. The disease affects more females than males and increases in frequency with age until at least ninety years. There is not enough data to really know the incidence in people who live beyond the ninth decade.

The exact cause of Alzheimer's is unclear but four genes and a blood protein known as ApoE4 have been linked to the disease. In addition, it is believed that smoking increases the risk. As part of the disease process, abnormal lesions, known as neurtic plaques and neurofibrillary tangles, form in the brain and the cortical area of the brain atrophies. As this happens, connections into and out of the brain are lost. Over time the ability to care for oneself and the ability to interact meaningfully with others and one's surroundings is lost. Alzheimer's patients are still able to move their arms and legs, but are clueless as to the rest of the world.

Alzheimer's affects the ability to perform daily activities and the ability to perform complex tasks. The first symptom is short-term memory loss. All of us suffer from this at one point or another. Who hasn't avoided introducing someone at a party because you can't remember his or her name? The difference is that people with Alzheimer's forget such things more often than not and never recall what was forgotten. Later symptoms involve other functions such as the ability to understand language and communicate the ability to perform purposeful movement, and the ability to be aware of surroundings and happenings. People with the disease find it hard to perform familiar tasks such as simple housekeeping. They have problems with language and may substitute unusual words for common items, making it difficult for others to understand what they are saying. They get disoriented as to time and place and frequently get lost in familiar areas. They have poor judgment and may dress or spend money inappropriately. Abstract thinking becomes difficult. They may no longer be able to perform simple arithmetic such as addition and subtraction. Things get lost, misplaced, or put in unexpected places. Mood swings are common as are major personality changes and lack of motivation.

You may be suffering from early Alzheimer's disease if you frequently experience any of the following:

▼ Inability to remember recent events such as appointments,

tasks, or assignments
▼ Trouble finding or speaking the right word
▼ Forgetting to do routine tasks such locking doors or feeding pets
▼ Forgetting how to use ordinary things like a hairbrush or pencil
▼ Failure to recognize familiar objects

Remember all of us are forgetful on occasion so you may not have the disease or your symptoms might be caused by a different illness. However, if you experience these symptoms, you should be evaluated by a physician. Bring a family member or close friend with you to the appointment so that the doctor can obtain a clear history of what has been happening. You might not be aware or able to remember how your daily activities are impacted.

Before the diagnosis of Alzheimer's can be made, your doctor will need to rule out other causes of dementia. Not all dementia is permanent or caused by Alzheimer's, although it is the most likely cause. It is important that the reversible dementias be tested for. Infection, inflammation, tumors, drugs, and nutritional deficiencies are examples of reversible causes of dementia. Testing will usually include blood samples and a brain scan in addition to a complete physical examination. Once the diagnosis of Alzheimer's is made, long-term planning becomes important. You want to make decisions about your future healthcare and finances before you become totally incapacitated. Do you want to be placed in a long-term care facility or do you have the finances to arrange for an individual caretaker? You may want to sign a living will or a durable power of attorney for healthcare and or finances. These kind of legal documents allow you to decide ahead of time what healthcare measures you want utilized to keep you alive. They also let you designate the person you would like to make your healthcare and/or financial decisions when you become incapacitated.

No cure for Alzheimer's disease exists. However, management plans have been developed to help ease the burden of the disease. Medicines are available that help somewhat with the cognitive loss and studies of newer medications are undergoing clinical trials. Behavior that is difficult to manage such as wandering, paranoia, combativeness, or resistance to personal hygiene measures like bathing can be helped with behavioral strategies and medications. Caregivers should talk to a doctor about the best way to cope. Make a list of the troubling behavior, when it occurs, how often it occurs, and what behavioral methods you have tried. Follow-up care is important. Your doctor should be alerted about any changes in symptoms and should be aware of other healthcare problems that can contribute to the dementia. An example of this would be an increase in hallucinations. The hallucinations may not be from progression of the Alzheimer's but rather caused by a urinary tract infection contracted from being incontinent.

The disease places a tremendous burden on the caregiver. The Alzheimer's Association has support groups all over the country and many local hospitals have educational programs that can help both the caregiver and affected individual. Ask your doctor what services are available in your area. You can contact the Alzheimer's Association at 800-272-3900 or visit their Web site at http://www.alz.org for more information.

## DISEASES OF TERRORISM
## (AN EVER CHANGING WORLD . . .)

September 11, 2001, and the months following have brought new medical challenges to the American people. Anthrax, a disease that most doctors only vaguely recall being mentioned in medical school, is headline news. We must now consider the possibility of a biological or chemical attack as a source of illness. When you consider the population of the United States, the mathematical probability is extremely small that any given individual will be a victim of this kind of terrorist action. However, the possibility exists and should not be ignored. The Centers for Disease Control and other public health agencies feel that biological agents that pose the greatest risk to the public are those that are easily spread or transmitted, frequently result in death, will probably cause public panic, and require special action for public health preparedness. The most likely diseases in this category include anthrax, smallpox, plague, botulism, tularemia, and viral hemorrhagic fevers.

## Anthrax

Anthrax occurs naturally in hoofed animals such as cows and is caused by the spore-forming bacterium *Bacillus anthracis.* The disease is not spread from person to person. Prior to the recent outbreaks, it was thought that it took being exposed to about 4,000 to 5,000 spores to cause infection, but that number is now in question. There are three forms of anthrax: inhalation, cutaneous, and gastrointestinal. As the name indicates, inhalation anthrax occurs when the spores are inhaled through the nose. The cutaneous form of the disease occurs when spores enter the body through a cut or opening on exposed skin. Gastrointestinal anthrax occurs when meat contaminated by the spores is eaten. Symptoms of the disease usually occur within a week of exposure and are similar to the flu. Cough, fatigue, fever, muscle aches, nausea, vomiting, and diarrhea are common. In the recently diagnosed cases, a runny nose was not a symptom. A sore may be present, especially on the face, arms, and hands. The sore is painless and develops a black scab surrounded by red tissue. Several antibiotics are available which can successfully prevent and treat the disease, if treatment is started early enough. In addition, a vaccine is available to prevent disease in people at high risk of exposure.

There is no screening test for anthrax. The Public Health Department uses nasal swabs and other testing methods to determine the extent of exposure in a given building or space but not to diagnose the disease. The diagnosis of anthrax is made when *Bacillus anthracis* is isolated from blood, skin lesions, or respiratory secretions of ill individuals or specific antibodies are found in their blood. Definitive testing for the disease can be accomplished in about one hour.

## Smallpox

Smallpox is caused by the Variola virus and it can be spread from person to person. Most people get sick within two weeks of exposure. Symptoms include high fever, fatigue, headache, and backache. A rash consisting of small blisters that can fill with pus occurs two to three days after the onset of symptoms. Smallpox can be confused with the common childhood disease chickenpox, but the pattern of the rash is different. In smallpox the rash occurs all at once and is located primarily on the face and arms, whereas a chickenpox rash starts on the trunk and develops over several days. Up until 1972, the United States required routine immunization against smallpox but it is not known if that vaccination will still be protective. Vaccination within four days of exposure will lessen the severity of the disease. Once you have started to have symptoms of the disease, it is too late for vaccination. Only supportive treatment, not drugs, is currently available for smallpox. The United States does have an emergency supply of the vaccine available and has already started vaccinating public health investigators.

## Plague

Plague is a disease primarily found in rodents and fleas that can infect humans. It is caused by the bacterium *Yersinia pestis*. It can be spread from person to person by face-to-face contact through respiratory droplets. A severe pneumonia develops that is fatal unless treatment is started within a day of onset of symptoms. Illness occurs one to six days after exposure. Symptoms include high fever, malaise, weakness, painful lymph nodes, and a cough with bloody or watery sputum. Several antibiotics are available to treat the disease and provide prophylaxis for those exposed.

## Botulism

Food-borne botulism occurs when a toxin made by the bacterium *Clostridium botulinum* is ingested in contaminated foods. Fear of this toxin is why you are advised to throw out any canned food with a bulging top. It is not spread from person to person but everyone who eats the contaminated food will get sick. Symptoms usually start six to thirty-six hours after eating contaminated food but may take longer. The first symptom may be blurred or double vision. Slurred speech and difficulty swallowing will follow. Eventually paralysis, starting at the top of the body and working its way down, occurs. Your shoulders will become weak before your upper arms. Your upper arms will become weak before your hands, and so on. An antitoxin is available to treat those affected with the disease and it works well in most cases. In addition, a vaccine exists to prevent the disease for those at high risk. A concern exists that, as a biologic weapon, the toxin would be inhaled rather than ingested, which would lead to greater exposure and more rapid onset of the disease. The impact of inhalation on the treatment of the disease is unknown. Incidentally, it is a botulism toxin, Botox, that is currently in vogue as a treatment for wrinkles.

## Tularemia

Tularemia was studied by both the United States and Japan for use as a weapon during World War II. It is a highly infective agent, requiring as few as ten organisms to cause disease. Inhalation of *Francisella tularensis* causes a febrile illness associated with pneumonia. The disease occurs naturally in the United States, primarily in rural areas. Every state except Hawaii has reported a case. The disease lives in many animals including mice, squirrels, and rabbits. It is not transmitted from person to person. Illness occurs three to five days after exposure, and symptoms include fever, chest pain, and enlarged lymph nodes. Early treatment with antibiotics is effective and antibiotics can be given to prevent the disease after exposure. A vaccine exists but is still investigational.

## Viral Hemorrhagic Fevers

Viral hemorrhagic fevers are a group of illnesses caused by distinct families of viruses. The illnesses caused by them may be mild or life threatening. The viruses live in animals such as rodents and insects like mosquitoes. A person can become infected by coming in contact with the saliva, urine, or feces of the animal or by being bitten or crushing the insect. Once infected, a person spreads the disease to another individual through close contact or contact with infected body fluids. Symptoms vary depending on the individual virus but most will cause muscle aches, fever, fatigue, and dizziness. Flushing of the face and chest may occur and there may be bleeding under the skin. No cure exists, so treatment is just supportive. Newer antiviral medications are being tried as treatment in several of these infections. Vaccination is available to prevent illness for some of the viruses in this group.

## Chemical Agents

Chemicals that might be used by terrorists range from known warfare agents to toxic chemicals used every day in industry. New chemicals are constantly being created, so it is difficult to specify exact preventive and treatment measures. A gas mask may not help you. Used incorrectly, a gas mask can cause death by suffocation. Gas masks were designed to be used *prior* to entering an area known to have toxic fumes. No warning will be given in a terrorist attack. The gas will just be released as it was in the Japanese subway attack a few years ago. You may very well succumb to the agent before you can get to your mask. If you suspect a gas attack, hold your breath, and head for the nearest open window or well ventilated area. If feasible, help those incapacitated around you. Not all chemicals used may be in the form of a gas. Liquids and oils may be released or sprayed directly into crowds. If this happens, use whatever is available to wipe it off your skin. Forget modesty and removed saturated clothing. As soon as possible wash vigorously with soap and water. Medical advice will be needed to determine the next steps you should take. The Centers for Disease Control is a good resource for additional information on specific chemical and biologic agents. The easiest way to access it is to search their Web site at http://www.cdc.gov. If you are unable to find the information you need, you can call 800-311-3435.

It is not a good idea to buy antibiotics just in case something happens. Don't put your doctor in the embarrassing position of having to tell you no. Public health agencies will make sure that all exposed individuals will be given the appropriate preventive measure when needed. The incorrect and indiscriminate use of antibiotics leads to bacterial resistance among microorganisms, causing common infections and increasing the risk of having a serious adverse reaction to them. Microbial resistance could well render antibiotics useless in a real attack or when you need them for an illness. Also, stockpiling antibiotics may rapidly deplete existing supplies and preclude access to drugs needed for normal purposes. Finally, taking antibiotics before a diagnosis is made may prevent or delay your doctor from figuring out what is really wrong with you.

You need to understand your own personal risk of being attacked by evaluating your place of employment, the sort of work you do, and where you live. Develop an increased awareness of what is going on around you. Be alert to suspicious activity. Inspect your mail before you open it. Whenever you are in an area with crowds or confined groups, know where the exits are located. Can you find your way out of the mall's movie theater without lights? Develop a plan with your loved ones that includes a meeting place and a number to call and leave a message in the event of an emergency. How will you cope if power is lost for an extended period of time? You may want to consider updating your basic survival skills. Can you start a fire for cooking without a gas lighter? Your best defense is to stay alert and be prepared.

Each phase of life offers new challenges. As an empowered health-care consumer, you need to focus on lifestyle changes that will help protect you from the five major killers, heart disease, cancer, strokes, chronic obstructive lung disease, and accidents. (Table 4 lists the leading causes of death for various age groups.) Fasten your seat belt, exercise regularly, and make sure your diet is low in fat. Don't drink and drive or drink and participate in water activities. Don't indulge in bad habits such as smoking or drug abuse. Develop a sense of personal awareness, so you will pick up on the early symptoms of serious diseases and notice suspicious events. (See table 5 for a list of symptoms.) Make promoting your health a priority. It's your body and your health.

## TABLE 4.  LEADING CAUSES OF DEATH

| Disease | Symptoms | Preventive Measures |
|---|---|---|
| Heart Disease | **Childhood**<br>turning blue, failure to grow, difficulty eating | early prenatal care |
| | **Adult**<br>chest pain, shortness of breath, pain with walking | no smoking, exercise, low fat diet |
| Cancer | **Childhood**<br>fatigue, paleness, mass, limp, joint or bone pain | avoid toxins |
| | **Adult**<br>chronic cough, fatigue, mass, weight loss, change in bowel or bladder habits, bleeding | no smoking, exercise, low fat diet, obtain cancer screening |
| Stroke | **Adult**<br>Transient ischemic attacks, loss of sensation, visual disturbance, headache, loss of coordination, paralysis, confusion | no smoking, exercise, low fat diet, control blood pressure |
| Chronic Lung Disease | **Adult**<br>chronic cough, shortness of breath | no smoking |
| Accidents | **Adults and Children**<br>high risk behaviors | wear seat belts, helmets don't drink and drive, guard rails |

## TABLE 5.  WORRISOME SYMPTOMS AS THEY RELATE TO DISEASE

| Symptom | Risk Factors | Possible Disease* |
|---|---|---|
| Difficulty breathing<br>Poor eating<br>Failure to grow *in newborns* | No or late prenatal care<br>Exposure to smoke prior to birth<br>Toxic exposure prior to birth | Birth defect or<br>Metabolic disorder |
| Poor school or work<br>    performance<br>Abusive language<br>Frequent physical fights<br>Increased accidents<br>Poor impulse control | Drug abuse<br>Alcohol abuse<br>Gang membership<br>Gun in home | Homicide<br>or Suicide |
| Fatigue<br>Flu-like symptoms<br>Rash<br>Blisters on mucous<br>    membranes<br>Frequent infections | IV drug use<br>Unprotected sex<br>Multiple sexual partners<br>Tattoos and body piercing | HIV or<br>Sexually<br>transmitted<br>infections or<br>Hepatitis |
| Weight loss<br>Fatigue<br>Lump or mass<br>Nagging cough<br>Change in bowel or<br>    bladder habits<br>Blood in stool<br>Unusual bleeding<br>Sexual dysfunction | Tobacco use or second-hand<br>    smoke exposure<br>Heavy alcohol use<br>High fat diet<br>Little exercise<br>Family history of cancer<br>Prior history of cancer<br>Age greater than 50 | Cancer, especially<br>lung, colon,<br>prostate, or breast |
| Chest, arm, neck,<br>    or jaw pain<br>Shortness of breath<br>Unexplained sweating<br>Sudden weakness<br>    or loss of function<br>Severe headache<br>Confusion | Age greater than 45<br>Tobacco use<br>High blood pressure<br>High cholesterol<br>    HDL-low, LDL-high<br>Diabetes<br>Relative with the disease | Heart attack or<br>Stroke or<br>Transient ischemic<br>attack |
| Increased hunger<br>Increased thirst<br>Increased need to urinate<br>Weight loss | Overweight<br>Little exercise<br>Tobacco use<br>Relative with the disease | Diabetes |

*not all the possible diseases listed are associated with all the symptoms or all the risk the factors, nor are all symptoms of the diseases mentioned listed here

# EMPOWERMENT TIPS

▼ Develop personal awareness.

▼ Obtain recommended screening tests.

▼ Visit your doctor for persistent vague symptoms.

▼ Avoid smoking and second-hand smoke.

▼ Wear seat belts and helmets.

▼ Remember alcohol can cause accidents.

# CHAPTER 5

# HOW TO AVOID ILLNESS

## (Wash Your Hands Before . . .)

Remember Mom insisting that you take a bath, get a good night's rest, exercise, and eat well? She was right. Hygiene, rest, exercise, and diet are the building blocks of good health. Most of us would rather forget about these basics and just pop a "cure all" pill when the need arises. Although pills may claim to cure our problems, the potential for health "quackery" is high. Don't believe the ads that promise instant weight loss, bigger breasts, and better sex. Good health isn't something you swallow. You have to work at being healthy by using the basics outlined by your mother, even if she didn't follow her own advice. Do these things on a daily basis to help ward off various illnesses and promote a long, healthy life. As it has been said for years, an ounce of prevention is worth a pound of cure. The time to start caring for your body is now. Don't wait until you start "falling apart" or "feeling your age" to initiate the basic preventive health measures that in reality should be lifelong habits.

## BE CLEAN

Personal hygiene plays an important part in health. Frequent bathing washes off bacteria and viruses from the skin that can cause illness and odor. Fear of smelling bad inspires most people to bathe daily (deodorant can only do so much), but hand washing is too often neglected. Failure to wash hands often enough is even a problem among healthcare professionals in spite of overwhelming medical evidence that hand washing can prevent the spread of infectious disease.[1] Be suspicious if your doctor doesn't have slightly damp hands or those that appear dry from frequent washing when she greets you.

Many infections are given to one person from another by "fecal–oral transmission." What this means is that germs get on your hands from contact with stool and then you put your hands into your mouth, passing the germs into your body. For example, prior to eating lunch, you shake hands with Mr. X, who did not wash his hands after going to the bathroom. Mr. X has a mild case of diarrhea. His hands are covered with the virus causing this illness and he passes it on to you. Two days later you come down with diarrhea. Washing your hands after using the bathroom, after changing a diaper, after handling pet waste, after shaking someone's hand, and before you eat can prevent such transmission.[2] However, you need to wash your hands even more frequently than that. Wash your hands before you prepare any food to prevent giving your germs to those you serve. Immediately wash your hands whenever you know you have come in contact with infectious material such as having just wiped a child's nose, picked up a used Kleenex, or handled dirty laundry. If you wait, you might forget or inadvertently put your hands in your mouth for some reason such as chewing on a pencil or biting a fingernail. Been around someone suffering from a cold? Wash your hands. Many respiratory illnesses can be prevented by frequent hand washing.

When navy recruits were ordered to wash their hands at least five times a day, they got sick a lot less than when they didn't have to wash their hands that often.[3] Think about doorknobs. Why do surgeons wander around with their gloved hands in the air? They want to avoid contaminating their recently scrubbed hands by opening a door. In public bathrooms consider using your foot to open the door or grabbing an extra towel to use to cover the door knob. New antibacterial gels that do not require water or drying and prepackaged hand wipes are available to make hand washing possible when soap and water are not readily available. Consequently, there is no excuse for not practicing this simple, yet very important, preventive health measure. However, using newer antibacterial products to clean your house is overkill and could lead to the development of bacterial resistance among the normal household germs that can be controlled now by routine cleaning. Plenty of effective hand lotions and moisturizers are available to prevent skin dryness and cracking from frequent washing. Just apply the lotion at bedtime or more frequently depending upon the dryness of your skin.

Good hygiene practices also extend to your mouth. Your teeth and gums need to be cleaned on a daily basis just like the rest of your body. You don't have to lose permanent teeth with pregnancy or as you age. Those are myths. If you want to keep your teeth, keep your mouth healthy. Periodontal or gum disease is the major cause of adult tooth loss; three out of four people over age thirty-five have some form of it. Regular brushing helps prevent decay and gum disease. Besides brushing your teeth twice a day, you also need to floss. Flossing removes plaque build up between your teeth where your toothbrush can't reach.

Most people don't think about their teeth affecting the rest of their body, but they do. Scientists aren't sure why having bad teeth contributes to other illnesses, but gum disease is associated with an increased incidence of pregnant women going into premature labor, as well as people having strokes and heart disease.[4] Symptoms of periodontal disease include tender and swollen gums, bleeding gums, loose teeth, a change in the way your teeth fit together when you chew, and persistent bad breath. If you find you always need a breath mint, or have any dental-related symptoms, start brushing and go see your dentist. Just like eating an apple, taking care of your mouth might well keep the doctor away.

## BE RESTED

Do you get enough sleep? Good sleep is essential for emotional and physical well-being. Our biological clock is sensitive to daylight and darkness. In general, we are sleepiest during the dark, especially late at night, and most alert during daylight hours, although a less intense period of sleepiness occurs in the mid-afternoon. In other words, even if you are well rested, you will naturally feel sleepy or less alert after midnight and around one o'clock in the afternoon. Biologic sleep needs vary among individuals, across the lifespan, and in response to physiological challenges such as illnesses. However, the *average adult needs approximately eight to eight and a half hours of sleep* to feel rested and alert upon awakening. If you never wake up before the alarm, consider going to bed fifteen minutes earlier.

Most of us are familiar with the symptoms of not getting enough rest. Though we're wise enough to put our cranky children down for a nap, we ignore our own exhaustion and end up apologizing for "biting someone's head off," because we were tired. We are aware, moreover, that people have died from falling asleep at the wheel while driving. In addition to making us feel tired, affecting our mood, and impairing our performance, lack of sleep affects other body functions that are not so readily apparent. It is generally believed that lack of sleep affects our immune system, making us more susceptible to disease. If you catch every cold that runs through your workplace, perhaps you need more rest.

Make getting enough sleep a bigger priority in your life. Small deficits add up over time to an amount that one long night of sleep can't replace. As a general rule, you will sleep better if you go to bed and awaken at the same time each day. If you take naps and find you have trouble sleeping later, decrease your naptime, move your nap at least four hours away from your anticipated bedtime, or don't take them at all. Avoid drinking caffeinated beverages in the evening and smoking near bedtime, as both caffeine and nicotine are stimulants. Alcohol may make you drowsy so you can fall asleep, but it interrupts normal, restful sleep cycles, so don't use it as a sleep aid. Sometimes eating a heavy meal late at night will disturb sleep. Try to keep late night eating down to no more than a light snack. Regular exercise can promote deep sleep, but not if done within three to four hours of bedtime. Make sure your sleep environment is as comfortable as possible. Try to avoid excessive light and noise. You may want to invest in a fan or other appliance to mask noise that you can't control. If you practice these good sleep habits and still feel you aren't sleeping well, talk to your doctor. Much more is now known about sleep disorders. New diagnostic tests are available and nonaddicting medicines can be prescribed to help you get the rest you need. Besides, it is possible that you have a medical problem, such as the breathing disorder sleep apnea, that is preventing you from sleeping well and making you more susceptible to illness and accidents.

## BE FIT

Couch potatoes, pay close attention. Exercise is very important to staying healthy and increases your chances of living longer. Exercise has been shown to decrease the risk of many diseases including hypertension, heart disease, diabetes, and cancer, yet the majority of Americans don't get enough exercise. They might be surprised to learn that the amount of exercise needed to stay healthy isn't that much. Only thirty minutes of moderate-intensity activity at least five days a week or twenty minutes of vigorous-intensity physical activity at least three times a week is needed. You are considered to be exercising at a moderate intensity level if you can talk comfortably and still exercise. On a scale of one to ten, a moderate intensity level would be a six. Your exercise does not have to be in units of twenty to thirty minutes to count. Shorter bouts of exercise have similar health benefits if done at a moderate-intensity level and if the total daily accumulation is at least thirty minutes. On any given day, most of us watch significantly more television than twenty to thirty minutes. We certainly could afford to give some time to exercise. Consider exercising during your favorite show. You won't miss anything and you will improve your health.

To be successful in adding regular exercise to your daily life, you need to be practical. No one is going to do an exercise they dislike on a daily basis. Choose something you enjoy. Your activity does not have to be structured or take place at a sports club or gym to count. Turning on the radio and just dancing is considered exercise. Similarly, choose an exercise that you can do with minimum inconvenience. If you have to fight traffic for an hour to jog on a track, you won't go on a daily basis. Choose an activity or activities that you can do regardless of the weather. Many people use too hot, too cold, and too wet weather as an excuse not to exercise regularly. Your exercise doesn't have to occur first thing in the morning. Look at your daily schedule and find a time when you are consistently free. You want exercise to become a habit. If you choose a time when other activities are likely to interfere, exercise will be neglected.

In addition to scheduled exercise, think of ways to increase physical activity in your daily life. Take the stairs instead of an elevator, if it is fewer than five flights. If you have a good sense of balance and hold on to the rail, walk on escalators and moving sidewalks. Besides increasing your exercise, you won't be shoved by the person in a hurry behind you. Don't place items on the steps and wait for them to accumulate before making the trip upstairs. Permanently lose the TV remote control. Carry your own groceries to the car. There are hundreds of ways to increase your activity level without much effort.

It is important to use caution when starting an exercise program. If you are on heart medications, have a history of heart disease, or suffer from any debilitating disease, talk to your doctor prior to increasing your exercise. You want to make sure you understand any limitations you might have and adhere to any recommendations. If you haven't really exercised in years, you need to *start slowly* and gradually increase your level of effort over a period of days or weeks. Doing too much, too soon can cause injury to muscles and joints. Do some stretching activities to *warm up* your muscles before doing more vigorous exercise and remember to *cool down* afterwards. As a rule of thumb, breathe out with exertion and inhale with muscle relaxation. For example, exhale while rising up to do a sit-up and inhale when you are back down on the floor. Make sure to include flexibility and muscle strengthening activities. Both are important. Maintaining your muscle strength can mean the difference between being able to get up if you fall down or lying there until someone pulls you up. On the other hand, maintaining flexibility is critical for good balance and coordination. If you can maintain your balance, you're less likely to fall and run the risk of injury. Good flexibility also helps cushion your back against sudden jarring motions. Most of us hate the abdominal exercises we had to do in physical education class but strong abdominal muscles also help protect your back from injury. Lastly, weight-bearing exercise helps prevent osteoporosis, the loss of bone that can occur with aging. Weight-bearing exercise is just that. Your body needs to be supporting at least your weight. Swimming is not a weight-bearing exercise because the water is supporting your body. Some people like to carry one or two pound weights when they walk to increase the amount of weight-bearing exercise they are getting. In other words, not only should you exercise on a regular basis, you should make sure your exercise program includes a variety of types of exercise. Your goal is to protect all of your body, not just your heart.

After exercising, you may be a little tired or slightly sore. Exercise shouldn't be painful or leave you exhausted. If that is the case, you've done too much. However, even if you are still sore on your next scheduled exercise day, don't put it off. You may need to modify what you are doing or add some extra stretches, but continue to exercise. Otherwise you run the risk of getting out of the habit and only exercising on occasion.

Don't let age be an inhibitor. You are never too old to start exercising. Even people confined to a wheelchair can benefit from a regular exercise program. Most healthy elderly people report they have been active their entire life and still exercise. In fact, exercise promotes longevity.[5] Stop just thinking you need to exercise and get off that sofa.

## EAT WELL

Eating healthy does not have to be boring or tasteless. You can have anything you want at mealtimes as long as you practice *moderation* and have a regular exercise program. It is okay to splurge every now and then and eat something incredibly fattening or loaded with salt and preservatives. Just don't do it every day and try to limit your portion. If you make a point of eating healthy and exercising five days a week, you likely won't get in too much trouble over the weekend unless you're a total glutton or have some underlying disease that requires strict dietary control, such as heart or kidney problems.

What constitutes a healthy diet? The National Cancer Institute of the United States Department of Health and Human Services and the Produce for Better Health Foundation, a nonprofit consumer education foundation representing the fruit and vegetable industry, have teamed up to give Americans a simple dietary message. Their message is *eat five or more servings a day of fruits and vegetables* for good health. The serving may be fresh, frozen, canned, dried, or in juice form. Another way of looking at this is color. Eat five servings of brightly colored food a day. Fruits and vegetables with the most nutrients tend to be brightly colored. Think about red tomatoes, yellow bananas, orange carrots, dark green leafy kale, purple eggplant, and so on. What counts as a serving? It depends upon what you are eating. Roughly speaking, an averaged size piece of fruit, a half-cup of cooked or canned fruit, or six ounces of juice is considered one serving. For vegetables, one cup of raw leafy vegetables or a half-cup cooked is a serving. Cooked or raw, you should strive for five servings on a daily basis.

Diets rich in fruit and vegetables are known to have a positive effect on the cardiovascular system and the body's immune system, and probably also benefit the skeletal system.[6] In addition, this kind of diet is naturally high in fiber and low in fat.

It is hoped that by shifting part of your intake to more fruit and vegetables you will decrease your consumption of higher fat foods without having to think about it. Although some fat is necessary in the diet because fat helps the body store energy, insulate tissues, and transport vital substances in the blood, most Americans eat much more than they need. A healthy diet should have only 30 percent of the calories daily coming from fat. Choose leaner cuts of meat and remove the skin from poultry. Eat more fish and dried beans or lentils because they provide protein and are lower in fat. And, of course, start limiting the amount of fried foods you eat. Yes, they are delicious, but they are also loaded with fat.

Although fish is considered a healthy food, be aware that the EPA (Environmental Protection Agency) has warned pregnant women and young children against eating shark, swordfish, king mackerel, and tilefish because of mercury contamination. In addition, pregnant women and children are warned to limit consumption of freshwater fish caught by family and friends. Contact your local Health Department or local Environmental Protection department for fish advisories that are specific to your area. On the Web you can go to http://www.epa.gov/ost/fish for more information and links to all advisory programs and contacts.

Diets high in fat, especially saturated fats, are associated with an increased risk of cancer, heart disease, and stroke. To confuse the issue, there are different types of fat. Some are better for you than others. Saturated fats are found in meat and in dairy products like milk, cheese, and butter. Unsaturated fats are found in both animal and plant sources and are further divided into monounsaturated fats like olive oil and polyunsaturated fats like safflower oil. Unsaturated fats, whether mono or poly, are better for you than saturated fats because they tend not to adversely affect cholesterol levels. Trans fatty acids are formed when vegetable oils are processed or hydrogenated. Think of unsaturated fats as being the better fats to eat and saturated fats and trans fatty acids as being the less healthy fats to eat. Terms on ingredient lists such as "partially hydrogenated vegetable oil" or "vegetable shortening" mean those products contain trans fatty acids. If a food product contains trans fatty acids, double asterisks (**) will be found next to the saturated fat listing on the food label. The asterisks are the new way the government has chosen to alert consumers to the presence of this ingredient. The hydrogenation process prolongs shelf life as it helps prevent fat from going rancid. Consequently, hydrogenated fats are used extensively in the baking industry to preserve shelf life of packaged baked goods and by fast food chains for frying. Thus an item can be advertised as cholesterol free, made from or cooked in vegetable oil, and still not be a healthy choice because of the use of hydrogenated fats. Become a food label reader. Try to choose items that are higher in the better fats and lower in less healthy fats. For example, substitute olive oil or another monounsaturated fat for butter. Buy soft tub margarines or those that are labeled trans fatty acid free instead of stick margarine. Stick margarine usually contains more trans fatty acids and saturated fats than the newer soft tub margarines because of the way it is manufactured. In general, the softer the tub margarine, the more likely that the first ingredient is liquid vegetable oil rather than hydrogenated vegetable oil.

High fiber diets benefit the digestive system and the heart, and may help protect against cancer. Dietary fiber comes from plants, not animals, and is not digested or absorbed by the body. Consequently it makes you feel full without contributing calories. For example, hot air popped popcorn is a high fiber, low calorie food unless you add butter or another topping. Fiber comes in two forms, soluble and insoluble. Insoluble fiber such as cellulose is passed through your intestines relatively intact. This kind of fiber adds bulk to your stool. Soluble fiber such as pectin forms a gel when mixed with a liquid and helps lower blood cholesterol. Most Americans eat less than the twenty to thirty-five grams of fiber daily recommended by the U.S. Surgeon General. Easy ways to increase your daily fiber intake include not peeling cleaned fruits and vegetables, eating whole grain breads and cereals, and drinking juice that contains pulp.

Vegetarians will obviously not have any trouble meeting the recommended five servings a day of fruit and vegetables. However, the more food groups you exclude, the harder it is to get all the nutrients you need. It is important for vegetarians, especially vegans who do not eat any product of animal origin, to make sure they get enough vitamin $B_{12}$, calcium, iron, and zinc. These nutrients are found almost exclusively in foods of animal origin. Vegetarians should pay attention to food labeling and make sure they are eating enough foods fortified with these substances to meet daily requirements. Vegetarianism is becoming more and more popular among teenagers today, so parents need to advise their trendy offspring that a wide variety of vegetables and perhaps supplements are necessary for growth and development. A diet of soda, chips, and cheese pizza is not healthy.

There are additional benefits to eating five servings a day of fruit and vegetables. These foods are known to be rich in substances called antioxidants. Included in the antioxidant category are vitamin C, vitamin E, selenium, carotenoids, and other phytochemicals. The body uses antioxidants to protect against tissue damage caused by normal metabolism. In addition to being associated with lowering cancer risk, antioxidants are also thought to help protect against the formation of cataracts and macular degeneration of the eye, both of which cause loss of vision.[7] Antioxidants may also play a role in preventing neurological diseases involving memory loss such as Alzheimer's disease.[8] It is interesting to note that, besides fruits and vegetables, antioxidants are also found in cocoa powder. There is at least one study that suggests a diet containing some chocolate is beneficial to the heart because of its antioxidants.[9] Could it possibly be that chocolate is really a healthy choice?

Perhaps the best benefit of a diet including five servings of fruits and vegetables is weight control. By shifting consumption away from food containing higher amounts of fat, most people will lose weight or not gain weight. When combined with a regular exercise program, weight control becomes even easier. Since as a nation, we are getting fatter, and since obesity increases the risk for many diseases, eating right takes on even greater significance. Don't view eating five servings of fruits and vegetables as a new diet. "Diets" are temporary changes in eating habits that may yield temporary weight loss. You want to establish healthy eating habits for the rest of your life and seize control of your weight in the process.

Getting older does not have to mean getting fatter. There are many ways to calculate your ideal body weight as determined by insurance and governmental figures and charts. In practice, most of us were at our ideal body weight when we graduated from high school. You likely recall what you weighed then. Chances are if you currently weigh within a few pounds of that weight you have done a good job in maintaining yourself. If not, you probably need to shape up. Keep in mind that although you may weigh the same as then, your weight may have shifted to other areas of your body and a larger proportion may be in fat rather than muscle.

To lose weight you must burn more energy than you consume. In other words, you must eat fewer calories and increase your activity. A pound a week is sensible weight loss and has a greater chance of being permanent because this rate of loss usually involves sustainable changes in your habits. Shifting your consumption to more fruit and vegetables from chips and other processed snacks is an example of a sustainable change that could start the weight loss process. You may want to give up snacks entirely or drink a glass of water instead. It is not unusual for people to mistake thirst for mild hunger.

In addition to striving for five servings of fruits and vegetables, you need to make sure you are getting enough liquid in your diet. Water is the beverage of choice since it has no calories and no artificial sweeteners, flavorings, or preservatives. The fluoride found in most public water is an added benefit because it helps fight tooth decay. Water in America is considered safe, unless you are getting it from a well or stream, since public water supplies are treated with chlorine to kill germs. Although popular, it is not necessary to filter water from your faucet. Many home water filters remove only minerals and other chemicals that affect taste, not the bacteria that can cause illness. If your filter has a brass fitting, you may actually be increasing the amount of lead in your drinking water. In truth, the water from your faucet may be safer to drink than bottled water from an unregulated natural spring. To find about the quality of your home water supply, read the consumer confidence report that should be mailed to you annually by July 1 from your water supplier. If you do not get one, you may request it or go to the EPA's Web site to see if it is posted (http://www.epa.gov/safewater/dwinfo.htm). For more information about bottled water and home water filters go to the Web site of NSF International (http://www.nsf.org/water.html), a nonprofit company that certifies bottled water and products used to treat water.

You should drink six to eight glasses of liquid a day to help your body remove wastes and toxins. Your needs will change depending on the weather and your activity level. You can tell if you are getting enough liquid by looking at the color of your urine. Dark yellow urine means you should be drinking more. Whenever you are sick, you need to increase your fluid consumption. This is particularly true with upper respiratory infections when your body is making a lot of mucous. It will be easier for your body to expel the mucous if you are well hydrated. Tiny hairs called cilia are responsible for moving mucous out of the respiratory tract, and cilia function much more effectively when you are well hydrated. The next time you have a cold, be sure to drink enough water to make your urine clear in color. You will then find it much easier to blow your nose and clear your throat.

You definitely should not consume six to eight glasses of alcohol or caffeinated beverages a day, although they are liquids! Alcohol consumption is associated with an increased risk of various cancers. The risk increases with the amount consumed. On the other hand, a glass of wine a day has been shown to reduce heart attacks. The secret is moderation. Most studies demonstrating risk with alcohol had consumption levels above two drinks a day. Note that 1.5 ounces of 80 proof liquor, 12 ounces of regular beer or 5 ounces of wine is considered a "drink." A double scotch on the rocks counts as two drinks even if the glass is small. Similarly, once you get beyond two servings of caffeinated beverages you start to see adverse health effects such as an increased heart rate, tremors, anxiety, and insomnia. The beneficial alertness and increased memory seen with caffeine does not increase beyond what you get with one to two servings.

What about food you eat in restaurants and prepared foods you buy? How safe are they? Unless food is properly stored, prepared, and handled, it can make you sick. Everyone has probably experienced the absolute misery of food poisoning. You went to a party and some dip containing mayonnaise did you and several of your friends in. However, other illnesses can also be the result of contaminated food consumption. The range of illness can be from mild, self-limited diarrhea and vomiting to death from a toxic *E. coli 0157H7* infection. How do you protect yourself?

In a store, make sure the meat and fish you buy are fresh. Use your nose. Does the store smell clean or are you hit by a nasty smell when you enter the meat and seafood department? Look for the sell date on the package and make sure it is current. Does the meat, fish, or poultry glisten and look like it was just wrapped or is it dull and the container soggy and stained? Make sure the coolers and freezers feel cold. Don't buy a package of meat, fish, or poultry that feels warm to touch. Avoid buying frozen goods that are soft or covered with crystals, indicating that they may have undergone partial thawing. They probably won't harm you, but the quality won't be as good. If you live in a hot climate, be sure to have extremely perishable items like shellfish or chicken livers packed in ice. Put your perishable items in a cooler until you can get them home. In colder climates, take advantage of the weather and place your perishables in the nonheated spaces of your vehicle like the trunk.

Most local radio and television stations immediately alert the public when a product that was sold in local grocery stores has undergone a food recall. If you have purchased a recalled product, don't eat it. If you are not sure if a product such as ground beef has been recalled, you can go the Web site of the Food Safety and Inspection Service of the U.S. Department of Agriculture and look up all products that have been recalled within the last six months (http://www.fsis.usda.gov/OA/recalls/rec_intr.htm). They also have a hotline you can call with questions or to report bad food. The number for meat and poultry products is 1-800-535-4555; for seafood the number is 1-800-332-4010. To report problems with other food products such as a sugar coated roach in a cereal box, you need to contact your local Food and Drug Administration Office. Look in the government section of your phone book under Health and Human Services. The food recall hotline should not be confused with the various hotlines that have been established to help consumers thaw and prepare frozen turkeys safely. The government site for that sort of information is http://www.fsis.usda.gov/OA/pubs/tbthaw. htm.

Food quality in a restaurant is harder to determine. Individual state laws control the inspection and health rating system of restaurants. There is no one rating system like stars for hotels in Europe to tell you what to expect. An 85 in one state is not equivalent to the same score in another state. Many local newspapers publish the scoring system and the inspection ratings of local restaurants on a weekly basis and some cities post these results on the Web. However, most people don't use the health rating as criteria for choosing a restaurant, nor does Zagat's. So use your common sense. Look at the menu. Is it clean? The menu is the one thing a restaurant knows you will examine closely. If they care about cleanliness, your menu will be spotless. Check out the bathroom. Is it nasty? If they don't keep the patrons' bathroom clean, do you think the kitchen behind closed doors is any better? Use your nose and sniff the air. If the air is thick with smoke and grease, the place is likely unclean. Look at your food server. Does he or she have clean hands? Remember this person touches your plate and silverware. Pay attention to food temperature. Hot foods should be hot and cold foods cold. If they aren't, send them back. Proper temperature either kills or prevents the growth of germs. Lastly, order ground meat dishes cooked well-done. Ground beef needs to be cooked to a temperature of 155°F to kill bacteria. Save juicy hamburgers for times when you control the preparation. Some of the recent *E. coli* outbreaks could have been prevented by thoroughly heating the meat involved.[10] Don't let the glamour of the establishment fool you. Even fancy, expensive restaurants have been known to receive a poor health inspection.

To eat safe food in a foreign country or island, use the same guidelines. However, also beware of the water quality. Drinking contaminated water or eating food such as salad greens washed in contaminated water is a frequent cause of "traveler's diarrhea," or in Mexico, "Montezuma's revenge." Don't be fooled into thinking that adding alcohol will protect you or that ice is okay. Also don't forget to wipe the top of cans or bottles clean before you start drinking. When in a foreign land, until you can verify the safety of local water, it is best to follow the old adage for food and water, "boil it, cook it, peel it, or forget it." Note that "nuking it" wasn't included as an option. Microwaves don't kill bacteria. It takes sustained high temperatures to kill germs. The government provides information about the water supply in foreign places on the Web. Go to http://www.cdc.gov/travel and click on "safe food and water."

Should you take dietary supplements? In the United States, if you eat properly, the answer is probably no. The press talks about antioxidants, vitamins, and other supplements that are supposed to help ward off cancer. However, as more research is done in this area, it is becoming evident that supplements aren't as good as the real thing and can be harmful in some cases. Eating five servings a day of a *variety* of fruits and vegetables is the smartest choice. Although supplements aren't a substitute for a healthful diet, some people such as pregnant women, postmenopausal women, and people on restricted diets may benefit from taking moderate doses of certain vitamins and minerals. For example, folic acid supplementation during pregnancy helps prevent birth defects, and adequate postmenopausal calcium intake is important in preventing osteoporosis. Talk to your doctor about supplementation especially if you have food allergies or other health problems that limit your selection of wholesome foods.

## GET YOUR SHOTS

The basics of good health, hygiene, rest, exercise, and diet aren't all you can do to help prevent disease and maintain a healthy body. You need to keep your immunizations current. Immunizations were developed to prevent serious diseases that can affect large numbers of people. To simplify the very complex natural protection system of the body, when a person gets sick, the immune system of the body fights off the infection. As part of the fight, antibodies are created against the germ that causes the infection. The next time the body comes across that germ, the antibodies recognize and eliminate it before you can get sick. This is why you only get certain diseases once. However, as mentioned in the case of flu, a germ can change so that the immune system doesn't recognize it. In addition, your immune system can be overwhelmed by a germ. Thus you can get some illnesses more than once. Immunizations work in a similar manner. You are given a vaccine containing an inactive or a weakened live germ or particle of the germ. This causes your body to create antibodies against the germ. Even though you didn't get sick, the antibodies created because of the vaccination will protect you against that disease in the future. Vaccines produce different strength immune reactions so you may need a series of shots initially or you may need a booster shot every few years. If the immunization is based upon a live germ, it is possible that you can spread the disease to others for a period of time. Your doctor should warn you if a particular immunization makes you contagious.

In addition to individual protection, when a large group of people is immunized against a disease, they can't spread the disease to others. Consequently, they confer immunity to the nonimmunized by keeping them from being exposed to the germ. This is known as herd immunity. However, herd immunity does not offer any protection to an individual for some diseases because the disease is not contagious from person to person. For example, you get the disease tetanus from contaminated soil, not people. People associate tetanus with stepping on a rusty nail, but it is the dirt on the nail and the puncture type wound that makes this kind of injury prone to infection with the tetanus organism. Therefore, herd immunity is not applicable in the case of tetanus; the risk of exposure remains the same.

Children should be immunized during early childhood. Your baby needs many shots before the age of two. You can contact your county Public Health Department for a list of places you can take your children to receive free or less costly immunizations and well child check-ups. Most counties list a number you can call for information in the blue pages of your telephone book. Look for a department titled "family and child services" or something similar. Many programs exist to insure that all children receive the immunizations necessary to keep them healthy. To get into school your child will have to have these shots anyway so you might as well get them at the proper time, during infancy, and give your baby the best protection.

Immunization against disease isn't just for kids. Our school system does a good job of making sure children are immunized against common childhood diseases, but once you leave school, it is up to you to get the shots you need. Doctors sometime forget to ask their adult patients about immunizations because of the time allowed between shots or boosters. Periodically ask your doctor to review your immunization records to make sure you are current. Occasionally special immunizations are required for travel to areas endemic for diseases not common in the United States. Check with your doctor prior to travel to make sure you are protected before you go. Or you can find out what you need by typing in your destination at the Web site http://www.cdc.gov/travel. Discuss the recommendations with your doctor.

For both adults and children, it is better to get an immunization when one is well. Sometimes an immunization will produce a mild reaction or illness. If you or your child were already ill, it may not be clear that an immunization reaction is occurring. The risk of a serious complication from a vaccine is far less than the risk of a serious complication from the disease it was designed to prevent, but on rare occasions they do happen. Remind your doctor of any medications that you or your child are allergic to because allergies to certain antibiotics may cause a severe reaction to an immunization. For example, if you are allergic to the antibiotic neomycin found in the common nonprescription triple antibiotic skin ointment, you should not be immunized against chickenpox. Likewise, let your doctor know if you or your children have had an allergic reaction to an immunization. A life-threatening reaction is possible with re-immunization. To be safe, discuss any reaction you or your children have had to previous shots, even if mild.

If you suffer from any chronic disease, your immunization needs may be different from those of the general public. Be sure to ask your doctor if you need additional or fewer shots because of your illness. For example, if you suffer from AIDS, you should not be immunized against chickenpox. On the other hand if you have a blood clotting disorder you should be immunized against hepatitis. In addition, if you are pregnant or trying to get pregnant, make sure you tell your doctor before you get any immunization. Some shots could cause birth defects in the baby if given too close to conception.

Immunization schedules are constantly being revised as new vaccines become available and as diseases become a threat to the population or are considered eradicated. For example, smallpox, once a standard immunization, hasn't been vaccinated against in years because the disease was no longer considered a threat to the American population. However, in view of September 11, consideration is being given to restarting smallpox vaccination. Up to date immunization information can be found on the Web from the National Network for Immunization Information at http://www.immunization-info.org. For healthy, nonpregnant individuals, routinely recommended immunizations currently include those described in the following sections.[11]

## Just for Children

### Pneumococcal Conjugate

The pneumococcal conjugate vaccine prevents pneumococcal meningitis, a serious infection that can result in permanent brain damage. Children under the age of two are at greatest risk for this disease. Therefore this immunization is recommended for infants.

### Haemophilus influenzae Type B

A series of four shots are given during infancy to protect children under age five from Haemophilus influenzae Type B, a serious bacterial infection. Prior to the availability of this immunization many young children died from this disease. Infection with the bacteria can cause severe pneumonia and meningitis.

### Polio

A series of immunizations is given in childhood to prevent the once common paralyzing disease poliomyelitis (polio). It is not currently recommended for persons eighteen years or older.

## For Children and Certain Adults

### Measles, Mumps, Rubella

A single vaccination, in some cases, can immunize against more than one disease, as in the case of the measles, mumps, and Rubella (MMR) vaccination. This immunization protects against these common infectious diseases of childhood. A booster shot is usually given during adolescence. Adults born before 1957 are considered immune to these diseases because prior to this date immunization was not available and most children contracted these three diseases. They still have antibodies to fight these diseases. Do *not* receive this immunization if you are allergic to gelatin.

*Varicella*

The varicella immunization is typically given in childhood to prevent chickenpox. One to two doses are required depending upon age. It is recommended for susceptible adults, those who have not had chickenpox and weren't vaccinated in childhood. Do not get this shot if you are allergic to gelatin.

*Hepatitis A and B*

A series of two injections are required for immunization against Hepatitis A, an infectious form of liver disease commonly spread through the stool. This is the type of hepatitis you get from contact with an infected individual or by eating infected food such as raw oysters. The vaccination is recommended for children over the age of two who live in areas where the disease is common. In addition it is recommended for adults with certain other illness and those at risk because of their lifestyle, occupation, or travels.

Vaccination for Hepatits B requires a series of three injections to protect against this blood-borne form of liver infection. It is recommended for children, nonimmunized high-risk adults such as those who use illicit injectable drugs, and heath-care workers exposed to blood.

## For Both Children and Adults

*Tetanus, Diptheria, Pertussis*

The original series of injections to prevent tetanus, diptheria, and pertussis is given in childhood and then is followed with a booster shot every ten years. Tetanus, otherwise known as lockjaw, causes severe, painful muscle spasms and is often fatal. Any contaminated wound, big or small, puts you at risk for tetanus if your immunization is not current. In childhood, immunization against pertussis or "whooping cough" is included. This component of the vaccination is dropped later because pertussis is not a life-threatening disease in older age groups, although they are a source of spread of the disease to unvaccinated children. Diptheria is highly contagious and causes membranes to coat mucous surfaces, especially in the throat. This can result in obstruction of breathing, severe pneumonia, heart failure, and death.

## For Adults and Special Needs Children

### Influenza (Flu)

Given once a year to prevent the flu, this vaccine is available to anyone desiring to lower their risk of getting flu. It is recommended for individuals over age fifty and those suffering from a chronic disease. People who work or spend time around the sick and elderly, such as caregivers and healthcare workers, should also be immunized. Women who will be more than three months pregnant during flu season should ask about getting this immunization. Do *not* get this immunization if you are allergic to eggs.

## Just for Adults

### Pneumococcal Polysaccharide

The pneumococcal polysaccharide vaccine is given as a one-time dose to people over age sixty-five, to those suffering from a chronic disease, and to other susceptible groups to prevent the lung infection pneumococcal pneumonia. One booster vaccination five years after the first dose is recommended in special cases. As mentioned earlier, bacterial resistance with pneumonia is increasing, yet the number of people getting this immunization remains low. You are urged to ask your doctor about your need for this immunization.

*Lyme Disease*

A series of three doses is required for immunization against Lyme disease, a tick-borne infection that causes arthritis. It should be considered for people ages fifteen or older who live in areas where the tick is common and who participate in activities that put them at risk, such as hunting and frequent camping. Proper protective measures against tick exposure should still be used. The use of this vaccine in younger age groups is currently being studied.

*Meningococcal Meningitis*

During their first year of college, students who live in a dormitory are at greater risk of contracting meningococcal meningitis. Immunization requires only one dose but a booster may be needed every three to five years to continue protection. Several states have made this immunization mandatory for all incoming college freshman planning to live in dormitories.

## BE SCREENED

In addition to being immunized against disease, you also need to periodically undergo screening examinations in order to stay healthy. Although the annual complete physical is no longer felt to be medically necessary for healthy adults with no symptoms, certain screening tests should be performed on a regular basis. The tests that are needed depend upon your sex and your age. Although many tests are available to detect disease, only the tests that have been shown to make a significant difference in the outcome of a disease are recommended for screening. *This does not mean, on an individual basis, that a test should not be performed, but rather that scientific evidence has not proven that obtaining that particular test makes a difference to the health of the general population.* Your doctor may recommend extra screening tests for you. What you want to find out from your doctor is why she feels you need additional testing. Keep in mind that rec-

# TABLE 6. STANDARD SCREENING TESTS

| Screening Age | Condition | Test Needed | Frequency of Test |
|---|---|---|---|
| Newborn | Metabolic disorders | PKU, Thyroid, Hemoglobinopathy | Usually once |
| All ages | Obesity | Height and Weight | Periodically |
| 3–4 years | Visual difficulties | Eye exam | Once |
| Over 21 years | Hypertension | Blood Pressure | Periodically |
| Males starting age 35, Females starting age 45 | High cholesterol | Blood cholesterol | Periodically |
| Females 50–69 | Breast Cancer | Mammogram | Every 1–2 years |
| Starting age 50 | Colon Cancer | Fecal occult blood Sigmoidoscopy | Annually Every 5–10 years |
| Males starting age 50 | Prostate Cancer | PSA benefit and risks should be discussed | Periodically |
| Elderly adults | Sensory loss | Vision and hearing screening | Periodically |

ommendations for screening are constantly being updated and revised as new clinical studies are completed and new tests become available. Standard screening tests currently recommended by the American Academy of Family Physicians and the United States Preventive Services Task Force include those listed in table 6.[12]

As previously mentioned, there is currently no recommendation for routine screening for diabetes. However, medical research is finding out more and more about the disease and learning that damage can occur to the body prior to the onset of any symptoms. Also, the number of Americans coming down with adult onset diabetes is growing, probably due to the increase in availability and popularity of high fat convenience foods and the overall decrease in exercise. With this in mind, you certainly should consider being screened for diabetes every three years, starting at age forty-five, if you have a family member with diabetes, are overweight, or have had diabetes during pregnancy. Recently the American Association of Clinical Endocrinologists in association with the American College of Endocrinology stated that this screening age should begin at age thirty. They also recommend screening be performed on all people diagnosed with heart disease, high blood pressure, high triglycerides, or low good (HDL) cholesterol levels.[13]

## PROTECT YOURSELF

Staying healthy also requires using your head. Your doctor will recommend you take certain preventative measures based on observational data and good old common sense. Controlled clinical studies on humans can't be done on everything. However, based on animal studies and knowledge of what has happened to specific groups of people, researchers assume cause and effect in certain instances. For example, ultraviolet-blocking sunglasses are thought to help prevent the formation of cataracts and macular degeneration of the eye. Cataracts are opacities that occur in the lens of the eye and block the transmission of light. Macular degeneration is a disease of the retina where the light-sensing cells malfunction. Both contribute to vision loss in the elderly. Many studies using animals have shown association of these conditions with ultraviolet exposure. In addition, people who have undergone total body irradiation as part of disease treatment experience more cataracts than those in the general population. The association has not been totally proven but, because of these findings, you should wear sunglasses if you are going to be outdoors for any length of time. No harm comes from wearing them and they are cheap if you aren't brand conscious. Buy glasses that are coated to block both UVA and UVB rays for the best protection. Polarized sunglasses protect you only from glare, not ultraviolet light, so don't get confused. Usually there is a label on the lens or printing on the earpiece of the sunglasses that indicates the ultraviolet protection. Don't forget to protect your children. Sun exposure is cumulative over a lifetime so start getting them in the habit of wearing sunglasses now when they are playing outside.

Along the same lines, the use of sun blocking lotions and creams help prevent skin cancer. Try to cover all areas of skin that will be exposed to the sun. Don't forget the tips of your ears or your scalp. You have to consider how clothing shifts with movement exposing previously covered skin. To get the best coverage, apply your sun block prior to putting on your swimsuit or other clothing. Your sun block will be more effective if it has a chance to sink into the skin before sun exposure. Try to apply your block thirty to forty minutes before you go outside and reapply frequently, even if the label says it will last all day. Water, sweat, and rubbing against anything or anybody can remove sunscreen, even the waterproof kind.

What strength should you use? Use a product with an SPF (sun protection factor) of at least 15. This means if your skin would burn with 10 minutes of sun exposure, the sun block lets you stay out 15 times longer or 150 minutes without burning. Products with an SPF of 15 block 93 percent of burning rays. Products with a SPF of 30 block 97 percent of burning rays, so higher SPFs don't add proportionately greater protection. The short ultraviolet rays or UVBs cause sunburn. The long ultraviolet rays, or UVAs, penetrate deeper in the skin and are associated with the skin damage of aging. Both are associated with skin cancer. There is some evidence that avoiding sunburn, especially when young, may lower the risk of the skin cancer melanoma. Newer sunscreens contain chemicals that will block both UVB and UVA rays. Make sure your sunscreen provides dual protection.

Since ultraviolet exposure is cumulative over your lifetime and sunscreens don't protect you completely from the harmful effects of the sun, skin damage builds up over time even if you don't burn. Consequently, even with block, limit exposure to the sun. Avoid being out midday, 11 A.M. to 3 P.M., when the sun's rays are the strongest. Wear protective clothing such as a hat and shirt. Keep in mind that thin shirts, such as a cotton tee, don't provide much sun protection. The average tee shirt has an SPF of about 4. Clothing is now available with higher SPFs. This clothing usually can be found in sporting goods stores and is great for people who spend long periods of time outdoors. Baby clothes are also available in these sun-blocking fabrics. Since it is preferable not to use sunscreens on children under six months of age, protective clothing and shade-providing umbrellas can solve the problem of what to do with the baby on a beach vacation.

Remember you can get burned on a cloudy day. Clouds block light, but not the burning ultraviolet rays. In addition, you can get burned in the winter, so consider using moisturizers or cosmetics containing sunscreen on your face. If you insist on always having a "tan," consider using "sunless tanners" rather than tanning beds that can emit harmful ultraviolet rays. Newer formulations of "sunless tanners" are easier to apply without streaking and can produce a realistic looking tan. The FDA feels that the active ingredient in these products, dihydroxyacetone, is safe. It creates a darker skin tone by interacting with amino acids found on the surface of the skin. Be warned that, although you will look tan, or even if you are tan, the color does not offer your skin any protection from the cumulative damaging effects of the sun.

It is well known that mosquitoes, ticks, fleas, other pests, and rodents carry and transmit disease to humans. The spread of the devastating bubonic plague in the 1300s was aided by fleas living on infected rats that bit people. Much more recently the West Nile Virus has spread down the East Coast from birds and mosquitoes to people. Fortunately most human cases are mild or without symptoms. Wear protective clothing and use insect repellant when necessary. Control the flea population on your pets so that your home and yard don't become infested. Keep lids on garbage cans and keep food products well sealed, so you don't offer an invitation to rodents to dine. Steel wool or screening tightly placed around pipe openings in walls and under sinks can effectively block entrances for creatures. Consult a professional exterminator if you have a serious problem. Remember the chemicals that you can buy for extermination purposes are poisons and must be used with caution and care. If you start feeling unwell after you have treated your house or yard, contact your local poison control center or doctor immediately. You may contact the American Association of Poison Control Centers free of charge at 1-800-222-1222 for information or to find the nearest poison control center. Of course, in any emergency when someone has stopped breathing, initiate resuscitation and call 911.

The evidence is not conclusive about a correlation between cell phones and brain cancer. It has been shown that genetic damage occurs when rats' heads are exposed to emissions like those from cell phones. In addition, studies that exposed human blood cells to these emissions also showed damage. It is felt that children under the age of sixteen are more susceptible to damage from cell phone emissions because their nervous system is still developing, their skull is thinner, and they have smaller heads.[14] Until the actual risk of cell phone usage has been determined (further studies are currently underway), you can lower your risk and your children's risk by using a hands free device or headset. Both of these devices keep the brain farther away from the antenna and the emissions. Furthermore, you will be able to keep both hands on the wheel when driving. You will still have to decide whether it is safe for you to talk and drive. The recommendation is to pull over and park, and some states, such as New York, are even beginning to legislate against using a cell phone while driving, unless a hands-free device is employed.

When participating in sports or when operating machinery, wear appropriate protective apparatus. Clearly many preventable injuries must occur if industry feels there is a market for the protection. Do you really want to spend a Sunday afternoon in the emergency room? Wear helmets and joint pads when roller blading, safety glasses when trimming weeds, and so on. It is well worth the effort to prevent just one accident. Similarly, if your balance isn't good and you're on rough terrain, use a cane or walking stick. Worried about falling or having a parent fall and breaking a hip? The Safehip is a device worn like underpants under clothing and may prevent a fracture. It has been proven effective in the nursing home setting.[15] Don't be lazy or vain, use the products designed to make your activities safer.

Be aware of your surroundings and environment and plan accordingly. Always know where the emergency exits are located. Know the fire evacuation plans for buildings you are in. Consider wearing 100 percent natural fiber clothing when traveling on an airplane. Natural fibers don't melt into the skin when they burn. In the event of a forced landing and fire, resulting burns may be less severe. In the winter, place a blanket in your vehicle for warmth while you await rescue, should you get caught in an unexpected blizzard. The blanket could protect you from severe frostbite. Likewise, carry extra water if you are crossing the desert on infrequently traveled roads. It takes much more time to starve to death but most of us can't go longer than three days without water. It goes without saying that you should always carry extra medicines with you that are vital to your survival. You don't know what may occur on any given day. Hopefully these situations will never arise, but take the time to be prepared.

## MAKE THE EFFORT

Breast-feeding helps protect against the later development of breast cancer in the mother. In addition, there is a growing body of evidence that demonstates multiple benefits for baby. It has been known for years breast-fed babies have lower rates of infections, allergies, asthma, hypertension, and other medical problems. Consequently, mothers are encouraged to breast feed their infants for at least six weeks, so that the baby will at least get the immune system benefits. It now appears that breast-fed babies may also be slightly smarter.[16] Although formula is an adequate source of nutrition, it does not contain everything found in breast milk. *Breast milk is the best* food for your baby, because it is tailor made. In fact, babies can distinguish between milk from their mom versus milk from others. Why not lower your breast cancer risk and have a healthier and possibly brighter kid? After all, breast-feeding is cheaper than formula and it doesn't have to be mixed, heated, or refrigerated.

Ever thought about having a pet? We don't know why owning a pet can be beneficial to your health, but data is beginning to show that, in addition to being wonderful companions (they don't talk back), pets actually promote longevity. It has been suggested that pets lower stress levels, decrease blood pressure, help prevent depression, and promote self-esteem.[17] Of course, you do have to keep your pet healthy. Pets and their waste matter can transmit disease. Talk to a veterinarian about what kind of pet is best for you and what health precautions you need to take, especially if you suffer from an immuno-suppressive disease. When your immune system isn't functioning properly you are more susceptible to catching a disease from your pet, so you want one that is disease free and easy to keep healthy. For example, you can get the disease Toxoplasmosis from cat feces. Normally this is a mild febrile illness like mononucleosis, but the illness can cause seizures if you are immunocompromised by AIDS. Pregnant women can pass toxoplasmosis on to the developing baby in their womb where it can cause great harm. Cats that play outdoors and eat raw meat are more likely to get Toxoplasmosis since the disease-causing parasite exists in the soil. You can prevent your cat from getting the disease by keeping it indoors and feeding it only dry or canned food. However, if you don't come in contact with your cat's feces, you can't catch the disease. The appropriate precaution is to wear gloves when cleaning the litter box and wash your hands immediately afterwards and/or keep your cat indoors and watch its diet.

Believe it or not, spirituality also impacts your health. Spirituality can be defined as your way of finding meaning, hope, comfort, or inner peace in your life. You may find this through religion, nature, principles, ethics, and beliefs; interactions with others, music; or perhaps through literature, or art. In some unknown way, the body and our psyche are connected. In addition to studies that have shown that a strong sense of faith improves surgical outcomes, it is well known that relaxation and meditation techniques can lower blood pressure and slow the heart rate.[18] Spirituality can promote hope and positive thinking in the wake of a medical crisis and help you cope with pain, fear, loneliness, and death. Take care of your inner self as well as your body. Make the time to do things that help you find tranquility. If you have spiritual concerns or beliefs that impact a healthcare decision, discuss this with your doctor. Your doctor understands the connection between the mind and the body and wants to encourage your well being.

## THE BOTTOM LINE

The principles of preventive health are very simple. The practice is much more difficult. However, what you do now helps determine the quality of the rest of your life. Take the time to establish good health habits now. Follow your mother's and doctor's advice, eat right, sleep well, get plenty of exercise, and take care of your body both physically and mentally. See table 7 for health-promoting goals and actions. For even more incentive to change your ways or encouragement to continue your healthy lifestyle, you can estimate your chance of living to a 100 by getting on the Internet and going to http://www.livingto100.com.

## EMPOWERMENT TIPS

▼ Practice good hygiene.

▼ Get enough rest.

▼ Make healthy eating choices.

▼ Stay active and lean.

▼ Take care of your body and mind.

## TABLE 7. HEALTH-PROMOTING GOALS AND ACTIONS

| Goal | Needed Action |
|---|---|
| Be clean and rested | Wash your hands frequently throughout the day<br>Floss and brush your teeth daily<br>Get 8 to 8.5 hours of sleep nightly |
| Eat well | No more than 30% of calories in diet from fat<br>5 servings of fruits and vegetables daily<br>6–8 glasses of water daily<br>Avoid excessive alcohol and caffeine consumption |
| Be physically fit | Maintain a healthy weight<br>Exercise at least 3 times per week<br>Do strength, flexibility, and weight-bearing exercises |
| Get periodic health check-ups | Keep immunizations current<br>Have recommended health screening tests<br>Be aware of and have unusual body changes evaluated |
| Be aware of your environment | Use sunscreen and wear sunglasses when needed<br>Protect yourself from insects<br>Always fasten your seatbelt<br>Use helmets, goggles, and other safety equipment<br>Get a headset for your cell phone<br>In buildings, know where the nearest exit is located |
| Enjoy life | Consider owning a pet<br>Stay in touch with relatives and friends<br>Participate in community activities<br>Take care of your inner self |

# CHAPTER 6

# UNDERSTANDING YOUR MEDICAL TEST RESULTS

## (Med School 101)

**M**ost doctor visits include some kind of testing. Not every test, as pointed out earlier, may be necessary. To avoid unnecessary testing and to gain insight into your own health and body, you need to understand what a doctor learns about you from common and frequently ordered tests. If you don't understand what vital organ or function a test evaluates, you will have a difficult time interpreting the results, even with an explanation from your doctor.

Note the word "interpret." Results of any medical test need to be taken in context. All medical testing is subject to interpretation. Most tests have a reference range or set of values that are considered normal for that specific laboratory and testing method, but any result falling outside this range may be perfectly fine based on other factors. For example, take your pulse. Put your fingers over the thumb side of your wrist or on your neck under your chin and count the number of beats you feel in a minute. If your heart is beating about seventy times per minute, your pulse falls within the reference range and is considered normal for an adult. If your pulse is lower than sixty, this can also be normal if you are in good physical shape. Similarly, if your pulse is over a hundred but you just carried three bags of heavy garbage to the street, it is still considered normal. The reference range needs to be used as a guideline, not an absolute measure of normal or abnormal. Interpreting results is not in black and white. Multiple variables and the possibility of laboratory or technician error need to be considered, too. Therefore, when given your results, do not panic because you have one abnormal test. The abnormal result may occur by itself or be an abnormal part of a panel, or group of tests. From a pure statistical point of view, the chance of a healthy person having one laboratory test result falling outside the reference range is 1 in 20.[1] The chance increases as more tests are run as a panel. In other words, without symptoms, you should view any single, isolated abnormal test with a healthy dose of skepticism. However, persistent abnormal or markedly abnormal tests may need further evaluation.

Medical testing can be accomplished in many ways but tests routinely ordered during an office visit usually call for easily obtainable specimens such as blood, urine, and stool. Many offices have a laboratory on the premises where medical personnel are capable of performing basic blood, urine, and other specimen testing. More complicated tests are sent to an outside laboratory though the specimen is still obtained at the doctor's office. Depending on the test ordered, where it has to be sent, and the location of the doctor's office, the results can be back in hours, days, or weeks. Doctors located in major metropolitan areas generally have greater laboratory services available and quicker response times than doctors practicing in remote rural areas.

## BLOOD TESTS (HEMATOLOGY, CHEMISTRIES, OTHER)

An easy way to understand commonly ordered blood tests is to look at what part of the blood is being measured. The blood contains white blood cells, red blood cells, platelets, and a great variety of chemical substances such as electrolytes, hormones, and fats. Blood tests can be divided into those that look at the components that make up the blood cells themselves and those that measure the chemical substances in the blood. The former are hematology tests and the latter are blood chemistry tests. For example, a test to see if you have enough red blood cells is a hematology test since it evaluates the blood cells themselves. A test to check your cholesterol level is blood chemistry test because it is measuring the amount of fat contained in the blood. Of course, many other kinds of tests requiring a blood specimen can also be ordered. Of these, ones checking to see if you have or are immune to a specific disease are the most common.

## Hematology

### CBC

Of the hematology tests, a *complete blood count* (CBC) is probably the most frequently performed. As the name implies, a CBC counts the number of red blood cells (erythrocytes), white blood cells (leukocytes), and platelets present. Red blood cells are essential because they contain the oxygen-carrying compound hemoglobin. White blood cells, of which there are five types, are important because they help protect the body against and respond to infection and inflammation. In other words, they fight germs and multiply when exposed to foreign substances, Unfortunately, in certain diseases they may even attack normal tissues of the body. Platelets form clots to prevent and stop bleeding. Too high or too low a level of any or all of these— red blood cells, white blood cells, and platelets—can signal disease. Your doctor will order a CBC to confirm or rule out the presence of a disease known to affect the blood make-up. This includes numerous conditions, both common and rare, such as infection, anemia, bleeding disorders, and leukemia. For example, red blood cell counts are typically low with anemia. White blood cell counts are usually high with significant bacterial infection and a low level of platelets can signal a bleeding problem. When only information on a single component is pertinent, individual tests can be ordered. Hence a doctor may order just a white blood cell count (WBC), a red blood cell count (RBC), or a platelet count. Results are given as the number of cells or platelets present in a specific volume of blood. Men typically have higher expected values than women. Values for children change as they move from birth to adulthood. Remember, reference ranges vary depending upon the laboratory and methodology used for performing the test. However, as a basic guideline, results falling within the following ranges are considered normal for adults:[2]

WBCs (white blood cells)   5,000–10,000/mm$^3$ both men and women
RBCs (red blood cells)   4.5–6.0 million/mm$^3$ men; 4.0–5.5 million/mm$^3$ women
Platelets   150,000–400,000/mm$^3$ both men and women

## Hg and Hct

Other frequently ordered hematologic tests are the hemoglobin (Hg) and hematocrit (Hct) tests. Both of these tests can determine the oxygen-carrying capacity of the blood. The hemoglobin test measures the actual amount of the hemoglobin present in the red blood cells blood while the hematocrit measures the amount of space or volume on a percentage basis that red blood cells take up in the blood. A hematocrit is sometimes referred to as a packed cell volume (PCV). Usually a doctor orders these tests to see if you suffer from anemia. Anemia is not the name of a disease but the name for a specific sign of disease. Consequently these tests don't say why you are anemic. They just verify it is present. The cause of the anemia can range from something simple like not getting enough iron in your diet (iron deficiency anemia), to having heavy menstrual periods (hemorrhagic anemia), or to having life-threatening cancer. As with other medical tests, the reference range for these tests is variable. Incidentally, erroneously low values can be caused by too much squeezing of your finger tip, causing dilution from tissue fluid. On the other hand, normal higher values are frequently seen in people who smoke.

Following are normal hemoglobin and hematocrit value ranges:[3]

Hg (hemoglobin)    14–18 gm/100ml males
Hg (hemoglobin)    12–16 gm/100ml females
Hct (hematocrit)    40–54% males
Hct (hematocrit)    37–47% females

If you only know one result, you can use the following formulas to quickly estimate the other factors:

$$Hb \times 3 = Hct$$
$$RBC \ (millions) \times 3 = Hb$$
$$RBC \ (millions) \times 9 = Hct$$

## Reticulocyte Count

The reticulocyte count is another common test of the blood components. The reference range for this test is .5–1.5 percent of total red blood cells or 25,000–75,000/mm$^3$.[4] Reticulocytes are immature or young red blood cells. Thus, this test really determines if your bone marrow is in good working order because both red and white blood cells are made in the bone marrow. Your body naturally increases the production of red blood cells in response to any significant blood loss. The loss may be from hemorrhaging or your blood cells being destroyed by some disease process. In either event, a healthy bone marrow will increase production of red blood cells and the reticulocyte count will be high. A normal or low reticulocyte count along with a low Hg or low Hct means that the primary cause of the anemia is due to the inability of the bone marrow to compensate for the blood loss. Further testing will be required to find out why the marrow won't respond. Any injury or disease that affects the bone marrow can affect the production of blood cells. However, depending upon the area damaged, only the production of red cells or all or some of the white cells may be affected.

## Peripheral Smear and Differential

In addition to measuring the number of blood cells present, sometimes the physical appearance of the cells is also evaluated. This test is known as a peripheral smear because blood is literally smeared across a slide and visualized under the magnification of a microscope. The size, shape, color, structure, and level of maturity of the blood cells and the platelets are evaluated since these characteristics have diagnostic significance in certain diseases. Results are given in terms of percentages of specific cells present and abnormalities seen. In larger laboratories, this test is now performed by very reliable machines. However, many smaller laboratories still perform this test manually, so the reliability of the results is directly related to the competence of the technician performing the test. A doctor usually specifies whether he wants the red blood cells screened, or the white blood cells, or both. A red blood cell evaluation is especially valuable in determining the underlying cause of any anemia that might be present. For example, if crescent shaped red blood cells pointed at one or both ends are found, sickle cell anemia is a likely diagnosis. On the other hand if the red blood cells have less color than normal or are hypochromatic, iron deficiency anemia is a more likely diagnosis.

The evaluation of the white cells is frequently referred to as a differential count, a diff, a leukocyte count, or a white cell morphology test because of the different kinds of white cells. Any disease or condition that affects the immune system such as infection, inflammation, allergies, hypersensitivities, drug reactions, and bone marrow and other cancers can affect the white cell count and differential. Each of the different white cell types (neutrophils, lymphocytes, monocytes, eosinophils, and basophils), serve a different purpose and the number of them present changes in response to both disease and physiological stress of any sort. The neutrophils, basophils, and eosinophils are frequently grouped together and called granulocytes because granules can be seen under the microscope within their cell matter. Neutrophils are the most common and account for 57 percent to 67 percent of the white blood cells.[5] They are critical to the body's protection against infection. Lymphocytes make up 25 percent to 33 percent of the white blood cells.[6] They play a big role in the immune process through the development of antibodies. Monocytes, making up 3 percent to 7 percent of the white blood cells, are one of the body's first lines of defense in chronic inflammation.[7] Eosinophils are active in allergic reactions and make up 1 percent to 3 percent of the white blood count.[8] Basophils are the least common. They make up 1 percent or less of the count and are important in nonspecific immune reactions to inflammation.[9] Based on the way your individual white cells respond and any shifts in their proportions as a result of stress to the body, your doctor can get a clue as to what is going on. The stress to the body can be anything. Your white blood cells react to both emotional stress, such as anxiety, and physiological stress, such as a fever. As a general rule, bacterial infections will increase your granulocyte count but viral infections increase your lymphocyte count. Based on your physical exam and your differential count, your doctor can reassure you that the cold you have had for a week is just a bad cold, not a more serious bacterial infection.

## ESR

The erythrocyte sedimentation rate (ESR) or sed rate is an excellent nonspecific indicator of inflammation. It is very sensitive to the presence of inflammation or tissue destruction within the body, but does not indicate where or what is the source. Just about anything can elevate an ESR. Consequently, it is not a good test to run unless symptoms of disease are present. It is particularly helpful in the diagnosis of rheumatologic diseases such as arthritis, diseases of the immune system such as AIDS, and in cancer. This test is also useful in predicting the severity of a stroke. Once a diagnosis has been established, the ESR may be used to monitor treatment and/or a reoccurrence. Because the test is nonspecific, elevations greater than 100mm/h usually indicate a serious underlying disease and will need further evaluation to find the source.

## Blood Type

Everyone wants to know his or her blood type. Nonetheless, no medical personnel will trust your word if they ask you for this information. The typing and matching of blood is so critical that all health-care personnel double check to make sure there are no errors. Also, many products exist to expand and help maintain your blood volume. These solutions, either a salt or crystalloid solution such as lactated Ringer's or a protein containing or colloid solution such as albumin, are readily available, can be given without typing, and are less expensive than blood. Consequently, blood is usually not the first fluid given when volume replacement is needed. Only under unusual and dire circumstances resulting in massive blood loss would unmatched blood be used. In the unlikely event that this is the case, you probably will be unconscious and unable to state your blood type. It takes a blood bank only fifteen minutes to type and cross match blood. Add another fifteen minutes for paperwork and transport time to and from the patient and the laboratory and blood can be ready in a half an hour. Therefore, your doctor will only use unmatched blood in situations so critical that he believes you won't survive thirty minutes.

Although many, many factors are checked to see if blood is compatible between a donor and a recipient, basically your blood will be one of four types: A, B, AB, or O (ABO system). The most common blood type is O and the least common is AB. Another important factor in the blood, especially for women of childbearing age, is the Rhesus factor (Rh factor). Your blood is considered negative or positive based on your Rhesus status. Most people are positive. When a woman is negative for the factor and her sexual partner positive, the potential for "sensitization" during pregnancy exists. Fortunately, the drug RhoGam was developed to prevent this. Prior to this drug, many women had "blue babies," babies that were born dead because the sensitization process caused the mother's body to destroy a positive baby's blood before it was born.

Type O negative blood is considered the universal donor blood because it is the safest type of blood to use when unmatched blood has to be given. Type O positive is the next best choice, especially for men, as they don't bear children and sensitization is not a concern. Unfortunately, O negative blood is not that common so people with this blood type are particularly encouraged to donate. Keep in mind that the term "blood transfusion" generally means the transfer of the blood or blood products. It is not specific for what part of the blood is being given. Only parts of the blood, such as just the red blood cells, the white blood cells, or the platelets in high concentrations, may be given depending upon the medical circumstance. If you require any sort of transfusion, you may want to ask what part of the blood you will receive. You should also ask if you can donate your own blood prior to any planned surgeries. That way you will have a perfect match, won't have to worry about catching an as yet unscreenable disease, and can lower your healthcare costs since you won't have to pay for the blood. However, even when your own blood is used, there are still fees associated with the collection, storage, and the actual transfusing of blood and blood products.

In case you want to know or would like to do a good deed, the best way to find out your blood type is to give blood. The American Red Cross can always use the donation and, as part of the process, you will find out your blood type. There is some evidence available that shows giving blood once every five years will reduce your risk of having a heart attack. Thus the life you save by giving blood may be your own.

As part of the donation process your blood will be screened for blood-borne diseases such as hepatitis and HIV to keep from contaminating the blood supply. Also at the time of donation, your blood is screened for certain antibodies. If you have these antibodies in your blood, you are likely to suffer from a serious reaction known as a transfusion reaction if you receive blood. This reaction can be prevented by using specially processed blood that most hospitals order ahead of time from a blood bank when it is known to be necessary. The Red Cross or another donation center will send you a card or otherwise notify you if you have these antibodies. Make sure to alert your doctor to this notification. This is especially true if you are scheduled for any type of surgery, no matter how minor. In the event you need blood in an emergency resulting from the surgery, it likely will not be available unless your antibody status is already known. This is good information to be put on an emergency medical identification necklace or bracelet along with any serious medical condition you suffer from, such as diabetes. (Necklaces are better than bracelets because they get noticed faster and are less likely to get lost.) Information about identification products can be obtained at most drug stores or you may want to visit the American Diabetes Association's Web site and view their buyer's guide for identification products at http://www.diabetes.org/diabetesforecast/2000Buyers Guide/pg60.htm.

For those who have ever had a blood transfusion, be aware that the FDA has started sending out blood recall messages. Obviously you can't give the blood back but you are being alerted to the fact that there might be a problem with the blood you received. The vast majority of these problems are theoretical in nature and not of clinical importance. For example, you may have received blood from a donor who traveled in England. Now that the medical community is aware of "Mad Cow Disease" and its association with the fatal dementia-causing illness Creutzfeldt-Jakob disease, blood received from anyone traveling to England can be considered suspect. The likelihood of this impacting your health is incredibly small. On the other hand, you may have received blood from an individual whose blood test for HIV did not seroconvert, turn positive, until after the blood donation. If you receive notification of a recall, you need to understand why the FDA felt the blood was a problem. Your doctor may not know where to get additional details about the notification. The most knowledgeable person in this situation is the pathologist in charge of the blood bank that gave you blood. Call the hospital and ask to speak to the doctor in charge of their blood bank or have your doctor call on your behalf.

## Blood Chemistries

### Electrolytes

Electrolytes are ionized salts found in the blood. Of these, sodium, potassium, and chloride levels are the most frequently measured. Perhaps the most worrisome electrolyte abnormality is an elevated potassium level. The upper limit of normal is 5.0 mEq/L but the individual response to a high level varies.[10] What your doctor fears is that an elevated potassium level will cause you to suffer from a fatal heart rhythm irregularity. A level above 5.0 mEq/L alerts your doctor that you are in danger and immediate corrective action must be taken. Common causes of elevated levels include such things as crushing injuries, heat stroke, and severely out of control diabetes. However, repeatedly clenching your fist after the tourniquet has been placed on your arm for blood drawing can cause an erroneously elevated potassium level, so avoid doing this. On the other hand, a low level of potassium (less than 3.5 mEq/L) is usually the result of prescription medication.[11] Diuretics used to treat hypertension and other illnesses are notorious for causing low levels. Under these circumstances, many doctors will prescribe potassium supplements or encourage their patients on diuretics to eat a banana a day to prevent this from occurring. Low levels can also be the result of illnesses such as food poisoning when you suffer from both vomiting and diarrhea. When you are afflicted with vomiting and/or diarrhea, it is important for you to maintain not only your hydration but your electrolyte balance. An easy way to maintain this balance is to pour an electrolyte-containing sports drink such as Gatorade over ice and take a small sip every fifteen minutes. Even if you are nauseated, you should try to drink at least a tablespoon every fifteen minutes to replace the electrolytes and fluid you are losing. Ginger ale or cola may taste better but they do not contain enough potassium. The stomach is capable of absorbing a tablespoon of liquid within fifteen minutes, so even if you have another episode of vomiting or diarrhea, chances are the drink will have stayed around long enough to be absorbed. Chugging a big glass of liquid all at once increases the risk of triggering an immediate response of vomiting. Stick to small sips until you have gone a few hours without running to the bathroom. It is hard to get children just to take one sip and wait. In this situation, you might want to make a popsicle by freezing a rehydration solution in paper cup with a spoon. Although your child might make a mess eating this popsicle indoors, it will prevent him or her from drinking too much too fast. Oral rehydration solutions designed for children under the age of two are readily available and come in both liquid and frozen forms. Again, with vomiting and/or diarrhea, it is important not only to replace the fluids lost but also the electrolytes. During flu season, it is a good idea to keep a bottle of a sports drink on hand just in case you get sick.

The electrolyte sodium is responsible for water regulation in the body. Most sodium abnormalities are caused when too much water is retained in the body as in congestive heart failure, or too much water is lost, as in dehydration. It also helps with the regulation of blood pressure. This is why many who suffer from hypertension need to watch the amount of table salt (sodium chloride) contained in their food. Sodium is found in all body fluids, including perspiration. Athletes in the South often take salt tablets prior to practicing in the heat to compensate for the sodium lost through the skin by sweating. They also drink plenty of fluids to replace the water lost. Your body is sensitive to changes in sodium levels. With just a slight increase in serum levels, you will feel thirsty. This is nature's way of protecting your electrolyte balance. Pay attention to your body and drink when you are thirsty. Many people ignore thirst, hoping to avoid a trip to the bathroom, and end up in the emergency room instead. Normal levels of sodium are between 135 and 145 mEq/L.[12]

Serum chloride levels are affected by the same conditions that affect serum sodium levels. Chloride levels usually shift in the same direction as sodium and to about the same degree. Hence, if the sodium drops, so does the chloride, and vice versa. There are a few exceptions. The most common is the low amounts of chloride that can occur with prolonged vomiting, although sodium levels may be relatively normal. In addition to its role in the electrolyte and fluid balance of the body, chloride is secreted in the gastric juice as hydrochloric acid and aids in digestion. The reference range for serum chloride levels is 96 to106 mEq/L.[13]

## Blood Fats

Most people probably worry about their blood fat levels more than any other test because of the clear association with heart disease and stroke. A fancy name for the test that measures your blood fats is a lipoprotein profile. To be most meaningful, this test should be drawn after fasting, at least nine hours without eating or drinking anything other than water. This profile will test for total cholesterol, both types of cholesterol, and your triglyceride levels. Each of these tests may be ordered separately but to get a clear understanding of your blood fats and your risk of atherosclerosis, you really need all the tests. Most doctors feel that your total cholesterol level should be under 200mg/dl. A total cholesterol level is the sum of all the cholesterol in your blood. However, you need to know the ratio of good to bad cholesterol in your body. Your HDL cholesterol, or high density lipoprotein, needs to be greater than 35mg/dl. Remember this is the "good" cholesterol because it helps the body remove cholesterol from your blood vessels. This is also the cholesterol that you can increase with regular exercise. Although 35 is a good level for your HDL cholesterol, a level of 60 or more is even better. Your LDL cholesterol, or low density lipoprotein, level should be less than 130mg/dl. If you already know you have heart disease you really need to get your level of LDL cholesterol to less than 100mg/dl. Even if you don't have heart disease, you want to get your LDL cholesterol as low as possible. If your LDL cholesterol level is above 130 after a three-month trial of therapeutic lifestyle changes to your diet and exercise habits, and you have other risk factors for heart disease, you should consider starting medication to lower your levels. Several classes of drugs exist to treat high cholesterol levels, including statins. Even though a drug of this class, Baycol, was recently withdrawn from the market because of the possibility of a severe reaction involving muscle tissue, statins are generally well tolerated and usually have few side effects. They have been shown to lower the incidence of heart disease and stroke by lowering cholesterol levels. Statins work by blocking the production of cholesterol in the liver. Remind your doctor periodically to evaluate the status of your liver if you are taking this kind of medication.

Triglycerides are the other fat in the blood. Your level of this fat should be less than 150mg/dl. The same healthy lifestyle that lowers high cholesterol levels also works to lower triglyceride levels. You may need drug therapy for levels higher than 150, especially if your LDL cholesterol is also high. Once you know your blood fat levels, you can go online to http://hin.nhlbi.nih.gov/atpiii/calculator.asp and calculate your ten-year risk of having a heart attack.

*Blood Sugar*

Glucose is formed from foods you eat during the process of digestion. It is absorbed by the small intestine and is stored in the liver as glycogen. Excess amounts are turned into fat and deposited throughout the body. Most cells of the body use glucose as a source of energy or fuel. The primary reason for ordering a glucose test is to screen for diabetes or to check up on the sugar control of a known diabetic. The reference range for a fasting glucose is 70–115mg/dl.[14] Levels of 110–125mg/dl are considered to reflect an impaired tolerance to glucose but not outright diabetes. Levels above 125mg/dl are in the diabetic range. As mentioned earlier, the diagnosis of diabetes is not made on a single abnormal blood glucose level. A low level of glucose in the blood is known as hypoglycemia and can result in mental confusion and even unconsciousness. This usually occurs as a result of poor diabetic control because the diabetic patient didn't match the amount of blood sugar lowering agent with food intake and activity level well enough to have a normal blood sugar level. It may occur in other circumstances such as exercising too long without having eaten. A glucose level of below 50mg/dl is considered in the hypoglycemic range. Early symptoms of hypoglycemia may include irritability, shakiness, blurred vision, sweating, and nausea. However, a rapid drop of glucose level, but not to the level of hypoglycemia, can cause similar symptoms. The treatment for hypoglycemia is to eat. This is why smart diabetics always have a nearby source of sugar such as hard candies or fruit juice.

*Liver Panel*

You can't live without your liver. The liver is responsible for many complex functions vital to life, including converting food to useable chemicals; making the substance bile, which aids in digestion; making blood clotting factors; and detoxifying the body. The liver is located on the right side of your abdomen just below your ribs. When a doctor pokes you in this area and asks you to take a deep breath, he is estimating the size of your liver. It enlarges and may become tender with certain diseases and conditions. Typically, when your doctor wants to check your liver, a blood test known as a liver panel is ordered. This panel includes more than one test because of the multiple functions performed by the liver, and because the substances that are being measured are not always exclusive to the liver. The tests measure damage to the individual liver cells and the ability of the liver to function. A liver panel consists of individual tests whose names are long and change as different assaying or testing techniques are developed. Once out of medical school, most doctors think and talk about liver tests only in terms of abbreviations. Without knowing the reference range of the laboratory used to run a liver panel, interpretation is difficult. You may want to ask your doctor for a copy of your test. The laboratory's reference range is usually included on the same sheet of paper as your results. In addition, individual tests on the panel need to be interpreted relative to the other test results. As a general rule of thumb, if there is no reason to suspect liver disease, a liver function test should be repeated before further evaluation is warranted and results should be at least twice the upper limit of normal to be particularly worrisome. This situation occurs when blood panels are ordered instead of individual tests. For example, you doctor wants to know your blood cholesterol level and your sodium level. Depending upon the laboratory used, the best way to get this information may be for the doctor to order a panel which includes liver function tests as well as the blood cholesterol and sodium levels. Following is a list of tests included in most liver panels and the significance of some results which may be cause for concern:

*Serum Aminotransfersases*—enzymes that act as sensitive indicators of liver damage. Their levels rise with liver cell damage but the degree of elevation is not a predictor of final health outcome. Your levels can be very high with a disease such as acute viral hepatitis and you can still make a full recovery.

▼ *AST or SGOT (Aspartate Aminotransferase, Glutamic-Oxaloacetic Transaminase):* This enzyme is found primarily in the liver and heart but also occurs in other parts of the body. Very high levels are often seen with acute hepatitis.

▼ *GGT or GGTP (Gamma-Glutamyl Transferase):* This enzyme is sensitive, but not specific, for gall bladder or pancreatic disease. Elevated levels are often found in people who habitually use alcohol because it is broken down by the liver. When compared to other enzyme levels, it helps distinguish whether elevated levels of other enzymes are coming from liver or bone. This comparison can help a doctor decide whether or not a cancer has metastasized to the bone.

▼ *ALT or SGPT (Alanine Aminotransferase, Glutamic Pyruvic Transferase):* This is an enzyme found in the liver and in lesser amounts in the kidney, heart, and muscles. Levels will start to increase with liver damage before levels of bilirubin (see below) are high enough to cause noticeable jaundice or yellowing or the eyes and skin.

*Albumin*–this is a protein that is made in the liver and its production is sensitive to liver damage. Low levels may be a sign of liver injury. The kidneys need to be functioning for albumin to stay in the blood so low levels can also indicate kidney problems.

*ALP or AP (Alkaline Phosphatase)*–this enzyme is found in the liver around the bile ducts and in developing bone. It is elevated when the bile ducts are blocked and when cancer has spread to either the liver or bone.

*Bilirubin*–this is a pigment found in the bile formed by the breakdown of the hemoglobin found in the red blood cells. High levels cause a yellowish cast to the skin known as jaundice. Elevated levels can be the result of too many red blood cells being destroyed, the liver not functioning properly, or, rarely, Gilbert's disease, a nonserious hereditary condition that results in higher than normal bilirubin levels with normal liver function. If you know you have Gilbert's disease, make sure you tell your doctor to avoid additional testing.

*Total Protein*—this is a measure of all the protein in the blood. It reflects the ability of the liver to perform its basic function of making protein for the body. Protein is a basic building block for the entire body. Thus a low total protein level is a sign of malnutrition. High levels generally are the result of dehydration or another cause of decreased body fluid volume.

## Kidney Tests

The *blood urea nitrogen (BUN)* is a test that reflects kidney function. Urea is made in the liver and excreted or eliminated from the blood by the kidneys. With normal liver function, the BUN test can be a good estimate of kidney function. Normal levels are less than 23mg/dl.[15] People with elevated levels are said to have "azotemia." Causes of azotemia can be divided into three categories: prerenal, renal, and postrenal. If blood flow is decreased to the kidney, creating an elevated BUN because not enough blood was able to be filtered of its urea, the cause is prerenal. If the filtration mechanism of the kidney itself is damaged the cause of the high BUN is renal. If urine is prevented from leaving the kidney, as with a kidney stone, the elevated BUN is from a postrenal cause. An elevated BUN shows only that there is a problem with the kidney clearing urea from the blood. It does not identify the cause of the problem.

*Serum creatinine* comes from muscle cell metabolism. Levels depend on your body muscle mass. The greater the muscle mass, the higher the creatinine level. Values for men typically are higher than for women. Creatinine levels also vary depending upon the time of day. Levels will rise after eating, especially after a meal containing lots of meat. A creatinine level is an indirect method of evaluating the kidney's ability to filter. However, depending on the method used, it may not be a very sensitive test. For example, having little muscle mass or being on a strict vegetarian diet could lower creatinine levels even though kidney damage was present.

*Thyroid Tests*

The thyroid gland might be considered the engine of the body. Its influence extends everywhere. It affects your heart rate, your cholesterol, your energy level, your mental state, your skin, and your muscle strength. Thyroid disease is relatively common, especially in women, but often is not diagnosed early. The single test most useful in diagnosing thyroid conditions is the TSH or thyroid stimulating hormone test. The pituitary gland of the body is responsible for telling the thyroid gland how much thyroid hormone to make. If the body isn't making enough, the pituitary encourages the thyroid gland to increase production by increasing blood levels of TSH. If the body has too much thyroid hormone, the pituitary gland lowers the level of circulating TSH, telling the thyroid gland to stop production. The normal reference range is 0.4 microunits to 4.8 microunits/milliliter of blood.[16] Low levels of TSH indicate hyperthyroidism. Symptoms of hyperthyroidism are those of increased metabolism, such as irritability, sleeplessness, heat intolerance, irregular menstrual periods, and weight loss. The most common type of hyperthyroidism is known as Grave's disease. Hyperthyroidism can be treated with drugs to lower the production of thyroid hormone, or with surgery or radioactive iodine to destroy part of the gland and thus limit production of the hormone. High levels of TSH are seen with hypothyroidism. Because the thyroid gland is being pushed by the pituitary gland to work harder, the thyroid gland often will enlarge with hypothyroidism. The enlarged gland is known as a goiter. Before iodine was added to table salt, hypothyroidism resulting from too little iodine in the diet was much more common. Symptoms of hypothyroidism are those of lowered metabolism such as fatigue, dry skin, mood swings, cold intolerance, and weight gain. Unfortunately, most of us need to blame our mouth, not our thyroid gland, for our weight problems. Depending upon the cause of the hypothyroidism, treatment may just involve taking daily thyroid hormone supplementation.

## Other Blood Tests

The number of blood tests available to a physician is enormous but, in the outpatient primary care setting, the most common other blood tests ordered by doctors are those that will identify a specific disease.

### Blood Culture

The blood culture is used to identify abnormal organisms such as bacteria that are growing in the blood. Typically a blood culture is obtained when you look very sick, have a high fever, and show no clear source of infection. If your temperature is 103°F, and your tonsils are swollen and covered with pus, a blood culture will not be necessary initially since the source of your illness is likely your throat. With infants, a high fever does not have to be present to warrant a blood culture. Any baby three months old or younger who has a fever of 100.4°F (38°C) or more probably needs a blood culture, and definitely needs a urine culture and very close observation with re-evaluation within twenty-four hours.

### Hepatitis Tests

The viral infection of the liver known as hepatitis is a common cause of abnormal liver panel tests. Other forms of hepatitis exist but types A, B, and C are the most common. Immunization against type A and type B was introduced in the 1990s, but none is yet available for type C. It is possible to be sick with hepatitis and not have any symptoms or have only mild ones. Many people inadvertently spread the disease, which is transmitted through contact with bodily fluids, because they don't know they have it. Consequently, May was named National Hepatitis month to increase public awareness of this serious and preventable disease. It is hoped that all high risk individuals will be immunized and that people in general will change their habits to reduce their risk of contracting hepatitis. A classic, hard to ignore symptom is jaundice or turning yellow. Other symptoms include headache, nausea, vomiting, weakness, fatigue, and abdominal pain.

In addition, urine may turn dark like the color of tea and stools may become unusually pale or gray in color. Smokers often report that they lose their taste for cigarettes.

Of the three, Hepatitis B and C are the most serious. Most individuals infected with Hepatitis A make a full recovery. Hepatitis A used to be referred to as infectious hepatitis because it is transmitted primarily through ingesting contaminated food, such as raw shellfish, and water. Good personal hygiene and proper sanitation helps to prevent Hepatitis A. On the other hand, Hepatitis B and C are transmitted by contact with blood or body fluids from an infected individual. The obvious source of this is intravenous drug use and having sex with an infected individual. However, body piercing and tattooing is also a risk for getting these types of hepatitis. Make sure only sterilized equipment and needles are used during these procedures. Manicures, pedicures, and haircuts with a straight razor also pose risk for transmission of hepatitis if the skin is broken and a solution capable of killing viruses have not been utilized between clients. Both Hepatitis B and C can progress to chronic hepatitis which may over time cause scarring or cirrhosis of the liver, liver cancer, liver failure, and death. Hepatitis C is the leading reason people undergo liver transplantation.

If your doctor suspects you may have hepatitis, she will want to find out what kind of hepatitis you have. The tests for hepatitis are designed to tell which type you have contracted and whether or not you are capable of infecting others with the disease. Normally, in response to disease, your body produces antibodies to protect you against foreign proteins or antigens. Once you have developed the antibody to hepatitis, you have it for life. You also develop these antibodies after successful immunization. It takes time to develop antibodies, so tests for the hepatitis antibody usually aren't positive until late in the course of the disease or one to two months after immunization. The time to develop antibodies varies from person to person so your doctor may have to repeat the test several times. Antigen tests are used to pick up the disease in the acute phase and when the virus is still present and you are still infectious. DNA tests are typically used to monitor treatment in people who develop chronic hepatitis. Your doctor will order the test or tests that are most appropriate for your stage of disease. Results are usually reported as positive or negative.

## Mono Test

Mononucleosis is a common viral illness that typically affects teenagers and young adults, although other age groups also contract the disease. It is caused by the Epstein-Barr virus (EBV). It is known as the "kissing disease," because transmission occurs by way of saliva. Many people who get the disease confuse it with other minor viral illnesses because symptoms are very mild in many cases. In its more serious form, it can affect the liver and spleen. Common symptoms include fever, a sore throat, fatigue, and swollen lymph nodes. Recovery occurs within days to several weeks, although some infected persons can take longer to fully recover. The disease is rarely fatal. There is more than one way to test for mononucleosis. The most common blood test is one that can be run rapidly in the doctor's offices. However, this test often may not show up as positive until late in the course of the disease so retesting may be necessary. More specific antibody tests to EBV exist and can detect the disease earlier. However, many doctors will make the diagnosis of mono, even with a negative rapid test, based on symptoms and the presence of atypical lymphocytes on a differential white blood cell count. In the past, the Epstein-Barr virus was also thought to be a cause of chronic fatigue syndrome but that has since been disproved.

## H. Pylori Test

As mentioned earlier, the bacterium *Helicobacter pylori* can cause peptic ulcer disease and it is associated with cancer of the stomach. There are many ways to detect the presence of this bacterium in the gastrointestinal tract but the blood test is perhaps the easiest. The bacterium can be detected in your stool, on biopsy of your stomach, or even from your breath. If antibodies to the bacteria are present in the blood test or another test is positive, you have *H. pylori* and should be treated with a course of antibiotics. Eradicating the bacterium from the body lowers your risk of recurrent ulcer disease. If you have been diagnosed with a stomach ulcer in the past and have never been tested, you should ask your doctor about this test. Additionally, if you live on antacids such as Tums or Rolaids or find yourself frequently taking over-the-counter Tagamet, Pepcid, or other stomach acid inhibitors, visit your doctor and request an *H. pylori* test.

## Syphilis

As long as people continue to have sex with more than one partner, especially unprotected sex, venereal disease will thrive. Many people catch a sexually transmitted infection with their first sexual relationship from a more sexually active partner. Although the discovery and use of antibiotics has lessened the impact of sexually transmitted infections, they still continue to be a major healthcare concern. Syphilis is caused by the bacterium *Trepoema pallidum* and is called the "great imitator" because the signs and symptoms of the disease can mimic so many other more "reputable" illnesses. It is a complex disease that has multiple stages. Initially a small, round, painless, firm sore or chancre may appear on the genitals, mouth, or elsewhere on the body. Left alone, the chancre will heal by itself in a few weeks. Next, a rash may appear on the soles of the feet, palms of the hands, or elsewhere on the body. This too will go away with time. Many years later, the organs of the body can be seriously compromised by the disease if it is left untreated. If you are at risk for any sexually transmitted disease (vaginal, anal, or oral intercourse) and notice an unusual sore, rash, or other symptoms, request testing from your doctor. As is true with most sexually transmitted infections, you can get syphilis more than once. There are several blood tests for syphilis. For screening purposes, most laboratories use the antibody-based tests VDRL test or the RPR test. These turn positive when you have the disease and remain positive for life even if you have undergone successful treatment. Before testing, advise your doctor if you have undergone prior treatment for syphilis so a different syphilis test can be ordered. In addition, it is possible for other conditions and substances to cause a false positive result. Don't accuse your partner of giving you the disease until your doctor has ordered confirmatory tests.

### Herpes

Herpes is a viral illness that can cause recurrent outbreaks of blisters around your mouth and genitals. The virus never leaves you although the interval between attacks becomes longer with time. You can spread this disease to others even when a blister is not present. Anyone with herpes should let any potential partner know they have this disease before starting a sexual relationship. "Cold sores" or "fever blisters" can be caused by the same strain of the herpes virus that causes genital herpes and vice versa. A herpes infection of the mouth or the genitals can be spread to either place depending upon the mucous membrane to mucous membrane contact. The diagnosis of herpes is usually made by the appearance of the sore and by a culture taken from a fresh blister. However, you may have a mild case and never notice a sore. The blood test, an antibody test, is useful when herpes is suspected but no sores are present to culture.

## URINE TESTS (URINALYSIS, CULTURE)

Urination rids the body of certain waste products. Produced in the kidneys and stored in the bladder, urine is usually pale to dark yellow in color, although certain foods can give the urine a different hue. Asparagus is notorious for not only turning your urine greenish but also giving it an unusual odor. Likewise, eating fresh beets can make your urine more reddish in color.

Tests on your urine can be used to screen or diagnose and monitor disorders of the kidney and metabolism, as well as infections. The most accurate and useful results come from properly obtained urine specimens. To get the best specimen, wipe your genital area clean and then start to void. Don't start collecting immediately. Void a small amount first, and then start to collect the specimen. This process is sometimes referred to as a midstream collection or a clean

catch specimen. It helps keep bacteria and other debris that might
have collected near the urethral opening from getting into the specimen and causing contamination.

## Urinalysis

The simplest, most cost-effective method to exam urine is with a dipstick. A strip of paper impregnated with reactants is dipped in your
urine and the resulting color changes indicate the presence or
absence of various substances in your urine, serving as an estimate of
certain bodily functions. Depending on the brand of dipstick used,
tests obtained and reference ranges will vary. The following can be
measured by using a dipstick:

▼ Ph–this is a measure of the acidity (acid) or alkalinity (base) of
   your urine. This varies depending upon the chemical balance
   within your body. Average ph for urine is 6.0.

▼ Specific gravity–this is a measure of the concentration of your
   urine. It reflects your hydration and the kidney's ability to reg-
   ulate water loss.

▼ Protein–this reflects kidney function. Normal protein loss by
   the kidney is up to 150mg/24 hours (dipstick reading of zero
   to trace).[17] Higher readings need further evaluation by
   looking at your urine under a microscope and/or by a quantitative urine protein measurement. Usually the protein found
   on dipstick is from a nonserious cause such as fever, infection,
   emotional stress, or intense activity.

▼ Glucose–sugar is not normally found in the urine. When it is
   present, an evaluation for diabetes is warranted. Diabetics
   who know they have the disease can monitor the control of it
   by checking their urine, although blood testing is more accurate.

▼ Ketones–this substance is normally not found in urine. It
   appears in the urine of people with poorly controlled diabetes, in those on extreme weight loss diets, and in those
   experiencing starvation.

▼ Nitrite—this substance should not be in your urine. Its presence is a marker for bacterial infection in the urinary tract. Some, but not all, bacteria that cause urinary infections produce this substance. Consequently you can still be infected even if nitrites are not found in your urine. Urine nitrite concentrations don't correlate with ingestion of products containing sodium nitrites as a preservative.

▼ Blood—the presence of blood is associated with urinary tract infections and a variety of other abnormalities, including bladder cancer. If infection is not the cause, evaluation of the urine by examination under the microscope is appropriate.

▼ Leukocyte esterase (LE)—the presence of this substance means that white blood cells are in the urine and suggests infection.

The dipstick is an indirect method to obtain information about your urine. Much of the same information and more can be gained by directly looking at your urine under a microscope. Because of this, the microscopic evaluation is used to further investigate abnormal dipstick results. A freshly voided, clean catch, midstream urine specimen is examined first with the naked eye for color and clarity. Cloudy urine is associated with extra cellular material which may result from infection. Abnormally colored urine may indicate an abnormal substance such as blood. The urine is then spun to separate out solid substances. A drop of the resulting sediment is placed under the microscope and evaluated. The substances that are seen, such as red blood cells (RBCs), white blood cells (WBCs), and organisms, are evaluated for type and quantity. Depending upon what is seen and the amount noted, a diagnosis may be made or further testing of the urinary system may be needed.

## Urine Culture

A urine culture is ordered to determine the identity of an organism causing a urinary tract infection. At the time of culture, sensitivities to antibiotics are also obtained. That way if the culture shows an infection, the doctor can place you on an antibiotic sensitive to, or proven to work against, the infecting organism. The standard of care for treating commonly acquired acute urinary tract infections based on either a dipstick or microscopic urinalysis is a three-day course of the combination antibiotic trimethoprim-sulfamethoxazole, providing no drug allergies exist. However, when infections don't respond to treatment or in the case of recurrent infections, the doctor should order a urine culture.

## OTHER COMMON TESTS (GENITAL, STOOL, STREP, PULSE OXIMETER)

### Genital

The sex organs are the source of much testing that goes on in a doctor's office. The genitals, unfortunately, are prone to trouble. In addition to routine Pap smears for women, any unusual discharge from either the penis or vagina and any discomfort with urination need to be promptly evaluated. Ignoring a discharge can lead to long term serious consequences such as infertility in either males or females.

#### Gonorrhea and Chlamydia

The test for the sexually transmitted infections gonorrhea (GC) and chlamydia can be done simultaneously using DNA probe testing. Typically a small swab is used to obtain some discharge from the cervical opening in the vagina or from the urethral opening in the penis. Sometimes a specimen is also obtained from the throat or anus. If either GC, or chlamydia, or both is found, you will need treatment with the appropriate antibiotics. The diagnosis of these diseases can also be made by culturing the organism or from a special urine test but many laboratories aren't equipped yet to run the urine test. Since the majority of people infected with chlamydia have no symptoms, the USPSTF recommends routine screening for this disease at the time of the annual Pap smear for all sexually active women aged twenty-five or under, and other asymptomatic women at increased risk for the infection.

## Wet Prep/KOH

This test is used to diagnose vaginitis. A sample of the vaginal discharge is placed on a glass slide and examined underneath a microscope. The chemical potassium hydroxide (KOH), is placed on half of the slide to remove cellular debris and make is easier to identify yeast cells. Based on the observed cells and organisms contained within the discharge, the kind of vaginitis may be diagnosed and appropriate medication prescribed. Many women recognize the symptoms of a yeast vaginitis and choose to treat themselves with an over-the-counter vaginal preparation. However, if you suffer from frequent infections or fail to respond completely to the medication you purchased, you may have misdiagnosed yourself. You need to visit your doctor and be evaluated. Frequent yeast infections may be the first sign of diabetes.

## Pap Smear

A Pap smear or Papanicolaou smear is a test that checks for cervical cancer. Early onset of sexual activity and having multiple sexual partners put women at risk for this kind of cancer. When treated early, cervical cancer can be cured. Moreover, conditions that are known to be precursors to the development of cervical cancer, such as the human papilloma virus (HPV), are recognized by Pap smear and can be treated before cancer has a chance to develop. A sample is obtained from the cervical opening in the vagina, preferably using a small brush like the one you would use to clean a bottle. The sample is smeared on a glass slide or placed in a special liquid to suspend the cells obtained. The newer method (Thin prep or AutoCyte prep) is the better way to perform a Pap smear as it can be more accurate. However, not all labs are set up to run the test this way and not all health plans will cover this more expensive form of testing. The laboratory results of a Pap smear should no longer be reported in terms of "class." That system has been replaced by the Bethesda and CIN grading systems. The new reporting system is an improvement because more information is obtained from the Pap smear. Information is given about the adequacy of the specimen received by the laboratory, as well as the presence of any infection or inflammation, the presence of any unusual or atypical cells, the presence of any growths, and the presence of cancer.

Based on these more explicit results, your doctor has a much better idea about the health of your cervix and will make appropriate follow-up suggestions. These may include repeating the test, being treated for an infection prior to repeating the Pap, or further evaluation by colposcopy. During colposcopy further diagnostic procedures such as a biopsy or a treatment such as freezing abnormal cells can occur.

## Stool

Like urine, fecal material is a waste product of the body and can provide useful information to your doctor about your gastrointestinal system and other parts of your body. For example, with phosphorous poisoning or hepatitis, the stool becomes pale or clay colored. Stools contain water, dry matter such as undigested cellulose, and a variety of other products such as bacteria and mucous. The most commonly ordered stool tests are used in the evaluation of acute diarrhea. As would be expected, a stool culture is ordered to see what type of bacteria is growing in the stool. A culture can't distinguish between normal *E. coli* bacteria found in the gut and the toxic strains of the *E. coli* bacteria. Consequently, when toxic *E. coli* is suspected, a special test, not readily available, to detect the toxin must be run. Viruses also can be the cause of infectious diarrhea. Many office laboratories are equipped to test stool for the presence of Rotavirus and Norwalk like viruses. The most common viral cause of dehydrating diarrhea in small children is a Rotavirus but older children and adults are more likely to be infected with a Norwalk like virus. To check for worms and parasites that might be causing a diarrhea, three separate stool specimens, a stool BOP test, need to be examined to see if the eggs (ova) or the creatures themselves are present. Three separate stool specimens means a sample of stool from three different bowel movements. You will not get an accurate test if you put part of one stool into the three different containers the doctor gives you. Other diseases such as irritable bowel syndrome and colitis may also cause diarrhea but the diarrhea is usually chronic. More extensive testing is required to make the diagnosis of that kind of bowel disease and treatment initiated.

### Strep

Most sore throats are caused by viruses, not bacteria. However, because strep throat is contagious and since tests to detect it are inexpensive, most doctors will make sure strep isn't the cause. Strep throat is caused by an infection with the *Group A beta hemolytic streptococcus* bacterium. Left untreated, it may result in long term complications such as rheumatic fever, which can affect the heart, or glomerulonephritis, which affects the kidneys. Strep throat is most common in school-aged children. However, many parents catch it from their offspring. You are considered contagious until you have been on antibiotic treatment for a full twenty-four hours. The diagnosis of strep can be made by a healthcare provider swabbing your throat with a soft tipped applicator and culturing the bacterium or performing a rapid reagent test. A strep culture takes about forty-eight hours to be completed. The rapid reagent test can be performed in a matter of minutes while you wait in the doctor's office. However, the test is not always accurate, especially if you have been sick for just a day. If your rapid test comes back negative, your doctor usually will double check the findings with a culture.

### Pulse Oximeter

The pulse oximeter is not a test in the traditional sense. The pulse oximeter is a piece of equipment that can measure how much oxygen is in your blood without a specimen having to be obtained. Usually the tip of your finger is attached to the device, which uses a beam of light to calculate the amount of oxygen in your blood. This test is frequently used to monitor asthma attacks and other respiratory conditions that might make it difficult to breathe. To give a good reading, the machine needs a good pulse. Hard, thick nail polish and fake nails can interfere with the machine's ability to detect the pulse and thus may prevent an accurate reading. Room temperatures cold enough to cause your blood vessels to constrict can decrease the pulse in the fingertips and cause an erroneous reading. If you are being monitored and feel chilly, request a blanket. The doctor or nurse may not realize you are cold unless you tell them.

## DIAGNOSTIC IMAGING (X-RAY, CT, MRI, ULTRASOUND, AND NUCLEAR IMAGING)

Tests that involve using specialized equipment and technology fall under the category of diagnostic imaging. Diagnostic imaging is used to view areas of your body that aren't otherwise visible. These tests may be enhanced by the use of swallowed or injected dyes. Imaging can also be performed in conjunction with another diagnostic procedure, such as when ultrasound is used to guide the placement of a biopsy needle. The imaging may be performed in the doctor's office as is common with X-ray and ultrasound, or at an out-patient testing facility or hospital.

The field of diagnostic imaging is experiencing rapid growth as new equipment and techniques are continually being developed. Old procedures are being replaced by newer, less invasive ones. For example, the small bowel can now be visualized by the M2A, a disposable capsule that is swallowed and excreted naturally, as compared to an endoscopic procedure where a physician inserts a tube with an attached camera through the mouth into the esophagus and stomach and looks directly. Swallowing a capsule is clearly more pleasant than endoscopy and it doesn't interrupt work or other daily activites.[18] However with imaging, the newest test is not always the best test for a certain problem. Your doctor has options when ordering a diagnostic imaging procedure. These include X-ray, CT, MRI, ultrasound, and nuclear imaging.

## X-Ray

The German scientist Wilhelm Roentgen discovered X-rays in 1895. He used X to describe them as X is the scientific symbol meaning unknown. To obtain an X-ray, radiation is passed through the body to a photographic film on the other side. X-ray tables have a place where the technician inserts the film in the form of a cassette. The denser a part of the body, the less radiation will pass through it. The less dense or softer body parts allow more radiation to get through to the film. Dense structures, like bone, appear lighter or whiter in color than softer tissues, such as an organ. X-rays are very good at diagnosing things like broken bones. The area of the bone that is broken provides a crack that lets radiation through. Consequently breaks can appear as dark lines on a white bone. The concern with X-ray is the amount of energy or radiation that is absorbed by the body. Newer technologies have been developed to keep this amount to a minimum.

Contrast material is a substance that blocks X-rays. It is used to make parts of the body appear clearer. For example, the gastrointestinal tract is soft and not very dense. Contrast material is swallowed before a series of X-rays is performed (upper GI series) so the tract will be more clearly visualized. In the case of angiography, contrast material is injected into an artery so that the blood vessel will be more clearly seen.

Multiple X-ray techniques, such as mammograms, have been developed over the years to visualize various structures within the body, and the techniques are continually being improved. For example, with digital mammography, a special electronic X-ray detector captures the image instead of a film cassette. The image is converted into a digital picture on a computer monitor. This allows the radiologist to adjust contrast and brightness and to magnify areas of concern for a clearer and closer look.

## CT

With Computed Tomography (CT), the X-ray tube surrounds the patient instead of coming in just one direction. Unlike X-ray where just one picture is taken of a part of the body, with CT multiple pictures are taken all at once from many directions. A computer takes the images and converts them into a two-dimensional cross section of the body part examined. Confusing and distracting images seen with traditional X-ray aren't present in a CT, which means a CT image can separate overlapping structures with great precision. Much more detail can be seen than with regular X-rays because CT allows for visualization of the soft tissue adjacent to bones. CT has become the imaging tool of choice in a wide variety of clinical situations, such as in viewing the sinuses in the head. Many facilities are offering full-body CT scans promising early warnings about serious disease. No studies have been done on the effectiveness of CT as a screening tool. Currently it is only approved by the FDA for diagnostic purposes on symptomatic or at-risk people. There is no evidence that having a total body CT will increase your longevity and there is a legitimate concern over the amount of radiation exposure involved with total body scanning and the risks involved with any subsequent follow-up testing. Before you agree to a total body scan, discuss any perceived benefits with your doctor. When CT first came out it was referred to as a "CAT" scan because only simple axial imaging was possible. It is now referred to as CT because, as the technology evolved, newer machines were developed capable of a multitude of images and computer reconstructions.

## MRI

Magnetic resonance imaging or MRI doesn't use X-rays, but rather employs a magnetic field and radio waves to create an image. You are placed within a tube and have to lie still so that a large, donut-shaped magnet can create the necessary magnetic field. Claustrophia, or the fear of small places, can be a problem with MRI. Open MRIs are available and can lessen this problem. If you feel uncomfortable in small places like an elevator, discuss this with your doctor so that your test can be arranged at a facility with an open machine. As with CT, a computer is used to process the information into a precise cross section of the human body. A distinct difference can be seen between normal and abnormal tissues. MRI is especially useful in imaging the brain, neck, spinal cord, soft tissues of the body, and joints.

## Ultrasound

Ultrasound imaging uses high frequency sound, or ultrasound, that is inaudible to human ears. A transducer, a microphone-like device, is placed on the skin over the area to be imaged and beams sound waves into the body. The amount of sound that isn't absorbed but is bounced back is measured and can be displayed as a two-dimensional image on a video screen. Ultrasound captures motion. This is very useful in imaging of babies before they are born and in studies of the heart and the heart valves. In fact an echocardiogram, or echo, is an ultrasound image of the heart. The echocardiogram looks at the structural health of the heart and its valves as compared to an EKG, which looks at the electrical health of the heart. When ultrasound is used to detect and monitor moving surfaces and fluids such as blood flow through a blood vessel, it is known as a Doppler study. Ultrasound has replaced traditional X-ray for some evaluations of the kidney, bladder, uterus, spleen, gallbladder, and pancreas. Ultrasound is not particularly good at imaging organs filled with gas or air, such as the lungs.

## Nuclear Imaging

PET or positive emission tomography scans and SPECT or single photon emission computed tomography scans use radioactive substances known as tracers to discern abnormal from normal structures and to evaluate body functions. Unlike X-ray, nuclear scanning develops images based on metabolism rather than anatomy. Consequently, it can best be used to study the function of a damaged organ or restriction of blood flow to areas of the brain. A tracer is introduced into the body where it gives off minute amounts of radiation. A special camera is used to detect the radiation and create the image. Different tracers are used to image different parts of the body. This kind of imaging is very sensitive and can pick up abnormalities early in the course of a disease. When tracers are combined with certain antibodies, the scanning is useful to check for reoccurrences of certain cancers such as prostate, ovarian, and colon.

Which test is best? This is a difficult question to answer. It really depends upon which body function or body part needs to be evaluated. As a rule of thumb, the test you want ordered will be the least invasive or risky and will provide your doctor with the most information. As an empowered healthcare consumer, before you sign a consent form for an invasive test, make sure you understand what the doctor hopes to learn from the procedure.

## EMPOWERMENT TIPS

▼ Reference ranges are a guideline, not an absolute.

▼ One abnormal test may not be significant.

▼ Understand what kind of test is being ordered.

▼ Ask what your doctor hopes to learn through testing.

# CHAPTER 7

# INTERNET SOURCES OF QUALITY HEALTH INFORMATION AND CARE

## (Click and Learn)

The Internet is leading the healthcare information revolution. Knowledge is not just power, it is empowering. Finally you have the medical world at your fingertips. You can search medical publications from around the globe. Nevertheless, you still need to be able to evaluate and interpret what you find. Not all Web sites are equal in quality and some aren't even remotely medically accurate. Just like on television, there are lots of commercials. You will be amazed at the supposed medical miracles that $29.99 plus shipping and handling will buy. There are no rules governing who can create a Web site or what they can post on it. You must decide if the information you find is reliable. To be on the safe side, always discuss what you have found with your doctor prior to taking any action that could impact your health.

## EVALUATING WEB SITES

The nonprofit organization Hi-Ethics was formed by representatives from the healthcare industry to help protect the healthcare consumer.

The organization is committed to insuring that healthcare Web sites contain trustworthy and up-to-date information, meet high ethical standards, and keep all personal identifying information private and secure. The principles established by Hi-Ethics were used by the American Accreditation Healthcare Commission (URAC) to establish an accreditation program for healthcare Web sites. URAC provides nationally recognized, neutral, independent, third-party assessments. Their program accredits sites that meet and maintain rigorous quality standards. To verify if a Web site is URAC accredited or in the accreditation process go to http://websiteaccreditation. urac.org. To date, thirteen health Web sites have received accreditation from URAC and can display the URAC logo. Clearly this logo, which is displayed below, will make it easy for healthcare consumers to recognize a quality healthcare Web site.

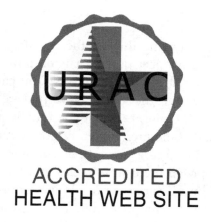

ACCREDITED
HEALTH WEB SITE

Along the same lines, Health on the Net (HON), a Swiss not-for-profit organization created by an international group of health professionals, promotes self-regulation of the Web by the health industry. To that end they have developed health Web site standards and an honor system for meeting these standards. Sites that display the HONcode logo meet their quality standards and are initially reviewed by the Health on the Net staff. Unlike the continual monitoring by URAC, it is up to the individual site Web master to maintain the standards after the initial review and up to viewers to report

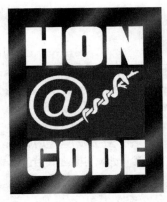

any violations. To learn more about this organization go to http://www.hon.ch/Global.

However, there are thousands of Web sites out there that don't feel the need to obtain any kind of accreditation. How do you judge these sites? To borrow again from Dr. George Lundberg's book, *Severed Trust*, there are five good rules to use in evaluating a health Web site. The rules, listed below, have been rephrased and explanations have been added that may slightly change Dr. Lundberg's intent. However the concept of the five rules is Dr. Lundberg's.[1] Many other people and organizations also offer similar criteria for judging Internet sites, but Dr. Lundberg was one of the first to publish the idea.

## Rule One: Who Is the Author?

You want to know the background of the Web site author or authors. Has the medical information presented been developed or reviewed by a doctor or professional staff from a reputable healthcare organization? Someone who works in the healthcare field should have access to more knowledge than someone who does not.

## Rule Two: Can You Contact the Site or the Author?

Contact information allows you to direct questions to the author to clarify anything you don't understand or to discuss the source of information. Your concerns about the validity of the information can be addressed. In addition, the contact address may reveal additional information about the origins of the site or the workplace of the author. For example, a contact address of someone@aol.com is more likely to be a self-proclaimed expert than doctor@St.Mary's-Hospital.com.

## Rule Three: Is the Medical Information
## Given Properly Referenced?

Knowing the source of the information gives you clues about its validity. Reputable medical organizations with a stated goal of public health education tend to provide very consumer friendly and accurate medical articles. Medical information obtained from reputable medical journals such as the *Journal of the American Medical Association* can be much more technical in nature because it was written with the healthcare professional in mind. On the other hand, although information from a tabloid may be more reader friendly, it should be verified by a reputable source.

## Rule Four: Who Funds or Sponsors the Site?

Many sites are designed to promote a particular product or sell health-related merchandise. Although some of the information on the site may be very good, claims about their products may be exaggerated. In other words, does the sponsor of the site have a reason other than the public good in giving you the information?

## Rule Five: How Old Is the Information?

You want the most up-to-date information. Medical information grows daily, especially in the fields of genetics and cancer research. Look and see when a Web site was last updated or posted. This is usually found at the bottom of a page. Look and see when a particular article was written. If the article is referenced, check and see if the sources used were up-to-date.

To help with these rules, you need to understand the types of Web sites that exist. As a rule of thumb, always look at the address, or URL, of the site you are visiting. By looking at the ending or domain (what follows the period, such as ".com" or ".net"), you get a clue as to the type of site you are visiting. The current main or "top level domains" are ".com," ".net," ".org," ".edu," and ".gov." As would be expected, commercial sites are generally ".com" or ".net." Organizations and charitable foundations typically use ".org." Academic institutions such as schools, colleges, and universities are usually ".edu." The government-sponsored sites use the ending ".gov." Keep in mind that as the Internet expands new domains such as ".info" are being developed.

Generally speaking, the most trustworthy health Web sites will be those sponsored by federal or state governments. These sites usually have the best interests of the healthcare consumer in mind. After all, your tax money is funding these kinds of sites, and the government wants to keep you healthy to decrease healthcare costs. National health organizations that represent medical conditions, such as the American Heart Association, or groups of physicians, such as the American Medical Association, are also very healthcare consumer oriented and very reputable. Academic and medical institutions are responsible for many sites on the Web. In general the information from these sites is excellent because they have their reputations to uphold. Pharmaceutical companies, the companies that make drugs, also sponsor Web sites. The information they provide about a medical condition is usually excellent, but keep in mind they probably will be promoting the drug they manufacture as the best treatment option. Sections of a managed healthcare plan Web site may be open to the general public. The information on these sites typically is geared to their membership and will promote services and products that are covered benefits. Since managed healthcare plans are structured to control healthcare costs, lower cost options may be discussed in greater detail than more expensive treatments. Sites promoting alternative and complementary medicine abound. Be very wary of the information found on these sites. If it sounds too good to be true, it probably isn't truthful. It goes without saying that sites created by individuals with no affiliation or sponsors are just that. Be skeptical of any health suggestion from a site whose only claim to fame is "it worked for me."

The best site for you of course, is the one sponsored by your doctor. Many medical practices now have their own Web site. In addition to information about the practice, on these sites you will find disease information that your doctor has screened and wants you to read.

Some individual physician's sites will also let you communicate with the office or doctor. You may be able to get test results or arrange for a prescription refill. The most wired practices will let you "virtually" see the doctor for specific simple, nonurgent problems. For example, you are going on a cruise and need the prescription patch to control sea sickness. Because you have a relationship with your doctor, a problem of this nature can be handled easily on-line. You may be required to pay in advance by credit card or give billing information before the site will send the message on to the doctor for this virtual visit or "Web visit" to the office. Typically the fees are less than those of a traditional office visit. Before seeking health information elsewhere on the Web, be sure to try your own doctor's Web site first.

Be aware that many healthcare information sites may also request personal information about you. For example, if you want to calculate your risk of getting a disease, use an on-line smoking cessation program, or track down a clinical trial for the latest cancer treatment, you will be asked to submit medical information that potentially could reveal your identity. You probably don't want the information you are submitting to be made public and linked to you. Consequently, before you submit any identifying information, make sure you read and understand a site's privacy policy. A reputable site will protect your privacy and give you a control over how your personal information is shared with others. Typically a link to the site's privacy policy can be found at the bottom of the home page.

Trust e is an independent, non-profit organization dedicated to protecting privacy and building user trust of the Internet. Sites that adhere to established privacy principles and agree to ongoing oversight may become members of the Trust e program and display the Trust e logo (above) on their site. To learn more about this privacy protection program or to verify the use of their "trustmark," click on their logo where displayed on a site or go to http://www.truste.com.

The wealth of information on the Internet is simultaneously one of the Web's biggest benefits and one of its biggest drawbacks. How do you find the best sites when so many are available? You may find that using multiple search engines will help you find exactly what you are looking for. There is a whole industry devoted just to getting Web sites to appear in the top ten listings of a search category within a search engine. Most of us will click on one of the first ten sites a search produces. In other words, depending upon the search engine you select, you will get different Web sites to choose from, even though you're searching on identical words or phrases. For example, using the search engine Yahoo! to search for "health" yields sites for the World Health Organization, CNN, the National Institutes of Health, the Department of Health and Human Services, and the BBC. The identical search using the search engine HotBot yields sites for the Lycos Network, the National Health Information Center, HealthWeb, the National Institutes of Health, and the government HealthFinder. If you are still having trouble finding the information you want, try the Google search engine located at http://www.google.com. Google uses a technique known as Web crawling where a computer searches the Web for new sites. Less commonly sought after information sometimes can be easier to find using Google. Incidentally, some of the better known search engines, like Yahoo!, use Google to provide some of the sites they list in their directories.

It takes time to search through all the healthcare sites that are on the Web and when you are facing a serious illness, sitting in front of a computer is probably the last thing you feel like doing. However, make the effort. Just taking control of your health and learning more about your condition will make you feel less helpless and may lead to a quicker recovery. Better yet, don't wait until you or a loved one gets sick. Start bookmarking healthcare sites that you find useful. Go beyond e-Bay and purchasing airline tickets on the Web. You will be amazed at all the interesting and useful health information you can find that can improve your day-to-day living.

## SUGGESTED SITES TO VISIT

Use the following sites to jump-start an individual, more extensive search. Keep in mind the previously mentioned rules to evaluating a site, and that the finance of Internet healthcare companies is in a constant state of flux. Although the sites are here today, they may be gone when you try to find them. Who would have thought a site with an ex-surgeon general of the United States behind it, dr.koop.com, would declare bankruptcy? On the other hand, new sites are being added. Dr. Tom Ferguson, a physician who has been writing about the empowered healthcare consumer and self-care since 1975, has an Internet site that periodically reviews new health sites and provides other information and links about health on the Web. You might want to sign up for his free online newsletter at http://www.fergu-sonreport.com. The sites that follow are organized under broad categories to make it easier for you to find what you need and want to know. They are listed in alphabetical, not preferential, order. All the sites mentioned are reputable and provide good information, although some are more technical than others. Each of us has different needs. Consequently you should bookmark the ones you find to be the "best."

## Warning Web Sites

Before listing some excellent Web sites, it is important to reiterate that *anyone can create a Web site.* Plenty of people have fallen for scams, especially health-related ones, on the Web. Because fraud is a problem, Web sites have been created to alert the healthcare consumer to the possibility. In addition, both of the sites listed directly below allow you to report any bad experiences. With policing, it is hoped the bad sites will be forced off the Web.

| Name | **Buying Medicines and Medical Products Online** |
|---|---|
| Address | http://www.fda.gov/oc/buyonline/default.htm |
| Author | Varies with selection |
| Contact | Multiple contact options available on the site |
| Source | Governmental agencies and institutions |
| Sponsor | U.S. Food and Drug Administration |
| Update | Given on articles |
| Highlights | Visit this site before you buy anything on line. Make sure you read the article entitled "How to Spot a Health Fraud." |

| | |
|---|---|
| Name | **Quackwatch** |
| Address | http://www.quackwatch.com |
| Author | Varies with selection |
| Contact | comments@quackwatch.com |
| Source | Stephen Barrett, M.D. |
| Sponsor | Quackwatch, Inc. |
| Update | Dates given on articles |
| Highlights | Informative articles and tips on how to spot and avoid medical fraud. Includes a listing and discussion of questionable medical practices and products. A version of this site is available in Spanish and other languages. |

## General Health Information Sites

The sites listed offer directories, medical dictionaries, encyclopedias, and links to reputable health information in a variety of forms and at a level that most healthcare consumers will be able to understand. Using these sites as an entrance, or portal, to the Web will allow you to find out basic information about disease prevention, diagnosis, and treatment. Following the links provided will take you deeper into the medical world and let you gain an even greater understanding of the disease process. There is no limit to what you can learn if you put your mind to it.

### Government Sites

| | |
|---|---|
| Name | **CDC Health Topics** |
| Address | http://www.cdc.gov/health/diseases.htm |
| Author | Professional staff |
| Contact | Multiple contact options available on the site |
| Source | Governmental agencies and institutions |
| Sponsor | Centers for Disease Control |
| Update | Given on selected article |
| Highlights | An alphabetical listing of diseases that is constantly being added to. This site also provides a link to other areas of the CDC. Much of the information is also available in Spanish. |

Name        **Health Finder**
Address     http://www.healthfinder.gov
Author      Varies with category selected but all have undergone professional review
Contact     dbaker@osophs.dhhs.gov
Source      Government agencies, non-profit organizations, universities
Sponsor     U.S. Department of Health and Human Services
Update      See individual sites
Highlights  A user-friendly site that will lead you to many reliable health information sources covering all aspects of medicine. Includes an excellent directory designed for finding information geared to your age, race, and gender. A version of the site is available in Spanish.

Name        **Medline plus**
Address     http://www.nlm.nih.gov/medlineplus
Author      Varies with selection
Contact     custserv@nlm.nih.gov
Source      National Institutes of Health and other reliable sources
Sponsor     U.S. National Library of Medicine
Update      See individual sites
Highlights  In addition to providing Medline, the tool to search scientific articles housed at the U.S. National Library of Medicine, this site has directories for other reliable health information, including current health news and fun interactive health tutorials. You can use this site to access the comprehensive medical encyclopedia created by ADAM.com, a leading originator of on-line health content and one of the first health information companies to receive URAC accreditation.

*Medical Organizations and Institutions Sites*

Name        **Family Doctor.org**
Address     http://familydoctor.org/

Author      American Academy of Family Physicians staff (physi-
            cians and patient education professionals)
Contact     email@familydoctor.org
Source      Varies with section selected
Sponsor     American Academy of Family Physicians
Update      Dates given on articles
Highlights  A collection of useful health information searchable by
            disease, body part, gender, or age. In addition, this site
            provides an excellent guide to self-care. A version of this
            site is available in Spanish.

Name        **Kaiser Permanente's To Your Health**
Address     http://www.kaiserpermanente.org/toyourhealth/index.
            html
Author      Professional staff
Contact     Multiple contact options available on site
Source      Material developed by Kaiser Permanente, the largest
            nonprofit managed care organization
Sponsor     Kaiser Permanente
Update      Home page updated daily
Highlights  Provides basic information about a variety of topics.
            The home page usually highlights a seasonal illness.
            There is a section of health tips designed especially for
            young children. This site will take you to Kaiser's *Health
            Information Check Up*, where you can find out the most
            popular health sites on the Web and see which sites their
            panel of experts recommends.

Name        **Medem**
Address     http://www.medem.com
Author      Member medical organizations
Contact     Telephone and e-mail contact information available on
            the site
Source      Member medical organizations
Sponsor     National and state medical societies
Update      Date given on articles

Highlights    The medical library on this site includes patient infor-
              mation from all of the sponsoring medical organiza-
              tions. This site also allows you to locate a specialty
              physician in your geographic area.

Name          **The Virtual Hospital**
Address       http://www.vh.org/
Author        Primarily from the departments of Family Medicine and
              Emergency Medicine of the University of Iowa College
              of Medicine. Bibliographies available on the authors.
Contact       librarian@vh.org
Source        University of Iowa College of Medicine with outside
              review by Mosby-Year Book, Inc.
Sponsor       University of Iowa Health Care, Mosby-Year Book, Inc.,
              Friends of Virtual Hospital
Update        Date given on different sections
Highlights    This is a searchable textbook of medicine for most
              common problems. You are encouraged to search the
              healthcare consumer or patient side first and then move
              on to the healthcare provider or professional side for
              more detailed information.

*Private sites*

Name          **InteliHealth**
Address       http://www.intelihealth.com
Author        Varies with selection
Contact       comments@InteliHealth.com
Source        Harvard Medical School Faculty
Sponsor       Aetna
Update        Home page updated daily
Highlights    Provides basic information about a variety of diseases
              and conditions. Has moderated chat rooms and discus-
              sion boards on many topics. On-line shopping is a fea-
              ture, so expect advertisements.

| | |
|---|---|
| Name | **Laurus Health.com** |
| Address | http://www.LaurusHealth.com |
| Author | Varies with selection |
| Contact | LaurusInfo@LaurusHealth.com |
| Source | Known public and private organizations, see list on site |
| Sponsor | VHA, Inc., a network of community-owned health systems |
| Update | Home page updated daily |
| Highlights | In addition to information about a variety of conditions, this site has a good section on healthy living. You may use this site to store your own health information and participate in interactive self-improvement programs. Advertising is a source of revenue for the site. |

| | |
|---|---|
| Name | **Medscape Health from WebMD** |
| Address | http://www.medscape.com |
| Author | Varies with selection |
| Contact | Multiple contact choices available onsite |
| Source | Varies with topic selected |
| Sponsor | WebMD |
| Update | Homepage updated daily |
| Highlights | The professional side of this site is used by many doctors to get up-to-date information. Includes medical news and reviews of journal articles. On the consumer side it has an "Ask the Experts" section which answers frequently asked medical questions about a variety of conditions and problems. Non–healthcare professionals may access either side. Required registration is free. |

| | |
|---|---|
| Name | **Praxis.MD Practical Answers for Patients and Physicians** |
| Address | http://www.praxismd.com |
| Author | Editorial board is supervised by Dr. Antonio Gotto Jr., Dean of the Weill Medical College of Cornell University |
| Contact | info@praxispress.com |
| Source | Clearly stated but varies with article |
| Sponsor | Praxis Press, Inc. |

| | |
|---|---|
| Update | Date given on all articles |
| Highlights | This is the home of the "Best Health Guide," a comprehensive and frequently updated consumer reference guide designed to quickly answer medical questions. It includes a Doctor Checklist that you can print out containing illness specific questions to ask your doctor prior to a visit. |

| | |
|---|---|
| Name | **Up to Date Patient Resources** |
| Address | http://www.uptodate.com |
| Author | Specialty physicians considered experts in their field |
| Contact | info@uptodate.com |
| Source | References given on all articles |
| Sponsor | UptoDate.com |
| Update | Every 4 months |
| Highlights | This site provides easy to understand, very sophisticated current information about a variety of medical topics. The site was started with the practicing physician in mind and recently added the consumer side. Access to the professional side requires a subscription but a free trial is available. |

| | |
|---|---|
| Name | **Veritas Medicine** |
| Address | http://www.veritasmedicine.com |
| Author | Biographies available on authors |
| Contact | info@veritasmedicine.com |
| Source | Many authors are faculty of the Harvard Medical School |
| Sponsor | Veritas Medicine |
| Update | Given on all articles |
| Highlights | In addition to providing solid information about various medical conditions including cancer, this site also provides data about new and investigational treatments. This site allows healthcare consumers to be matched to ongoing clinical trials on new treatments based on information submitted electronically. |

Name          **WellMed**
Address       http://www.wellmed.com
Author        WellMed professional staff
Contact       Multiple contact choices available on site
Source        Physician developed
Sponsor       WellMed, Inc.
Update        Updated regularly
Highlights    Free membership required to access a wealth of specific healthcare information. This site has many tools to calculate your individual health risk, check on your health status, and store and track personal health data.

## Cancer Sites

Cancer is the disease that sends many healthcare consumers to the Web looking for answers. The Web does offer a wealth of information about treatment options and can facilitate the enrollment in clinical trials for treatment that may offer new hope. Cancer can make otherwise rational people desperate and willing to try anything, even if it sounds crazy. There are people who prey on your having this kind of reaction to the diagnosis of cancer. *Before you commit yourself to any new or unconventional therapy, discuss it with your doctor.*

Name          **American Cancer Society**
Address       http://www.cancer.org
Author        American Cancer Society professional staff
Contact       Contact information, including telephone numbers, is available on site
Source        The American Cancer Society, which, incidentally, is the largest not-for-profit source of cancer research funds.
Sponsor       American Cancer Society
Update        Dates given on articles
Highlights    An in-depth resource for all types of cancer information. Free registration is necessary to access certain sections. The site contains a cancer profiling section that guides you through cancer treatment options and side effects

based on your specific cancer information. Included in the profile is a list of questions to print and discuss with your doctor. This site is a great start for anyone newly diagnosed with cancer.

| | |
|---|---|
| Name | **Association of Online Cancer Resources** |
| Address | http://acor.org |
| Author | Not applicable |
| Contact | Contact information available on site |
| Source | Varies with selection |
| Sponsor | Association of Online Cancer Resources |
| Update | Varies with selection |
| Highlights | This is a comprehensive listing of cancer-related support groups and Web sites. It currently gives access to 143 mailing lists, some of them in Spanish |

| | |
|---|---|
| Name | **Oncolink** |
| Address | http://www.oncolink.com |
| Author | Varies with selection |
| Contact | webmaster@oncolink.com |
| Source | University of Pennsylvania Cancer Center |
| Sponsor | List of sponsors available on site, primarily pharmaceutical companies |
| Update | Varies with selection |
| Highlights | Provides information on a wide range of both childhood and adult cancers. An interesting feature is the "Onco Tip" of the day. The site also provides a clinical trial matching service. |

| | |
|---|---|
| Name | **National Cancer Institute** |
| Address | http://www.nci.nih.gov/ |
| Author | Cancer experts |
| Contact | Multiple contact options available on the site |
| Source | PDQ database |
| Sponsor | National Institutes of Health |
| Update | Regularly updated |

Highlights   Contains a database (PDQ) that provides summaries on the most current information available on all aspects of cancer from prevention to alternative treatments. You may choose to read a nontechnical, patient friendly version or the one designed for physicians. Clinical trial information is given. The site is also available in Spanish.

Name        **Y-me National Breast Cancer Organization**
Address      http://www.y-me.org/english.htm
Author       Professional staff with resource credits listed
Contact      Multiple contact information available on the site
Source       Y-Me, a nonprofit organization founded in 1978 to offer support and counseling to those afflicted with breast cancer
Sponsor      Corporate sponsors listed on the site
Update       Dates given on various sections
Highlights   In addition to facts about breast cancer, this site provides emotional support for women diagnosed with the disease. It has a hotline available to answer questions about any of the materials presented. In addition, it sponsors a monthly teleconference with experts to about breast cancer topics for breast cancer survivors under the age of 40. The site is also available in Spanish.

## Heart Disease and Stroke Sites

As you know, more people die from heart disease than from any other illness. The factors that can lead to a heart attack also can cause a stroke. The following sites offer insight into the origin of heart and blood vessel disease and give updates on what is being done in terms of prevention, diagnosis, and treatment. Knowledge can empower you to live the healthiest lifestyle possible.

Name        **American Heart Association**
Address      http://www.americanheart.org
Author       American Heart Association professional staff

| | |
|---|---|
| Contact | Multiple contact options available on the site |
| Source | Professional organizations and resources |
| Sponsor | American Heart Association |
| Update | Date given on articles |
| Highlights | Very user friendly site designed to educate the public about all aspects of heart disease. Heart attack symptoms are clearly discussed with multimedia options. Healthcare consumers are encouraged to "act in time." |

| | |
|---|---|
| Name | **Cardiology Channel** |
| Address | http://www.cardiologychannel.com |
| Author | Professional staff |
| Contact | Information available on the site |
| Source | Material developed and monitored by board certified physicians |
| Sponsor | HealthCommunities.com |
| Update | Home page updated daily |
| Highlights | This site provides basic information specific to diseases of the heart. The information is often accompanied by useful illustrations. The site is trying to develop a community for visitors with cardiac concerns. Items are offered for sale on this site. |

| | |
|---|---|
| Name | **National Heart, Lung, and Blood Institute** |
| Address | http://www.nhlbi.nih.gov/index.htm |
| Author | Varies with selection |
| Contact | NHLBIinfo@rover.nhlbi.nih.gov |
| Source | Governmental agencies |
| Sponsor | Department of Health and Human Resources |
| Update | Varies with selection |
| Highlights | Includes many printable information sheets about diseases affecting the heart, lungs, and/or blood. Some of these are available in Spanish. |

| | |
|---|---|
| Name | **My Heart Watch** |
| Address | http://www.myheartwatch.org |

Author        Varies with section of the site
Contact       Contact information available on the site
Source        Varies with the section of the site
Sponsor       American Heart Association
Update        Given on the site
Highlights     This is a free personalized interactive health community program designed to educate you on heart attack and stroke prevention. You can calculate your heart attack risk and find out how to better the odds. You must enroll to get the benefits of the many features such as a health planner, a nutrition calculator, and an Ask the Expert section. This site is also designed to give support to caregivers of those suffering from heart disease and stroke.

## Lung Disease Sites

Since there is currently no cure for Chronic Obstructive Lung Disease, the Internet can be a great source of comfort and support for those who suffer from this condition. Research is ongoing. Perhaps you will find a suggestion your doctor feels would be reasonable for you to try. Of course COPD is not the only disease affecting the lungs. There are many other respiratory conditions and diseases of the lungs that are also addressed by the following sites.

Name          **American Lung Association**
Address       http://www.lungusa.org
Author        Varies with site selected
Contact       Multiple contact choices available on the site
Source        American Lung Association
Sponsor       American Lung Association, the oldest volunteer health organization in America. The members of their Board of Directors are listed on the site.
Update        Home page updated daily
Highlights     Has a fact sheet available on various lung diseases. Many of the articles are also available in Spanish.

Name        **The Health Library at Stanford**
Address     http://healthlibrary.stanford.edu/resources/internet/
            bodysystems/respiratory.html
Author      Not applicable
Contact     health.library@medcenter.stanford.edu
Source      Health Library at Stanford
Sponsor     Stanford Hospital and Clinics
Update      Not applicable
Highlights  Comprehensive listing of links to sites for specific lung
            conditions. Use the link back to the library home page
            to see resource lists on other conditions.

Name        **National Jewish Medical and Research Center**
Address     http://nationaljewish.org
Author      National Jewish professional staff
Contact     Multiple contact options available on the site
Source      National Jewish Medical and Research Center, a non-
            profit medical and research center devoted entirely to
            respiratory and immune diseases.
Sponsor     National Jewish Medical and Research Center lists their
            corporate sponsors and advertisers on the site
Update      Given on each article
Highlights  Contains a comprehensive selection of fact sheets on
            diseases affecting the respiratory system. They have a
            "lung line" where you can talk with a registered nurse to
            obtain specific answers about lung disease. A version of
            the site is also available in Spanish.

Name        **National Emphysema Foundation**
Address     http://emphysemafoundation.org/
Author      Foundation professional staff
Contact     gary@emphysemafoundation.org
Source      National Emphysema Foundation
Sponsor     Hinds Research Center
Update      Update given on articles
Highlights  Excellent educational material about the lungs. Contains
            a detailed section about how to keep your lungs healthy.

| | |
|---|---|
| Name | **Medline Plus** |
| Address | http://www.nlm.nih.gov/medlineplus/copdchronic obstructivepulmonarydisease.html |
| Author | Varies with selection |
| Contact | custserv@nlm.nih.gov |
| Source | National Institutes of Health and other reliable sources |
| Sponsor | U.S. National Library of Medicine |
| Update | See individual sites |
| Highlights | Includes an excellent interactive tutorial that clearly explains what goes on in the lung with the condition COPD. Some of the articles are available in Spanish. |

## Other Disease-Specific Sites

Although the threat of cancer and the health of our heart and lungs are foremost in most our minds, the rest of our body is important too. These sites focus on diseases involving other organs or body functions that are significant to our overall health and enjoyment of life.

| | |
|---|---|
| Name | **Alzheimer's Association** |
| Address | http://www.alz.org |
| Author | Professional staff |
| Contact | info@alz.org |
| Source | Alzheimer's Association, which sponsors much of the research in this area of medicine |
| Sponsor | Alzheimer's Association |
| Update | Given on articles |
| Highlights | This site provides in-depth information about this disease on a consumer and healthcare professional level. It also has a very useful glossary of terms related to Alzheimer's disease. |

| | |
|---|---|
| Name | **American Diabetes Association** |
| Address | http://www.diabetes.org |
| Author | Professional staff |
| Contact | Customerservice@diabetes.org |
| Source | American Diabetes Association |

Sponsor   Corporate Sponsors are clearly identified and mentioned on sponsoring sections
Update    Dates given on news articles
Highlights In addition to providing basic information about the disease diabetes and its relationship to diet and exercise, the site allows you to enter your zip code and find out about diabetes-related support services and activities in your area.

Name      **American Liver Foundation**
Address   http://www.liverfoundation.org
Author    Professional staff
Contact   webmail@liverfoundation.org
Source    American Liver Foundation, which funds medical research in this area of medicine
Sponsor   American Liver Foundation
Update    Given on the site
Highlights In addition to giving information about diseases of the liver and gall bladder, the site also provides links to ongoing clinical trials. More detailed information will soon be available along with a Spanish version of the site.

Name      **An AIDS and HIV Information Resource–The Body**
Address   http://www.thebody.com
Author    Varies with selection
Contact   Multiple contact options available on the site
Source    Varies with selection
Sponsor   List available on site, many pharmaceutical companies involved
Update    Given on all articles prior to linking to them
Highlights In addition to many articles on all aspects of HIV and AIDS, this site includes an interactive test where you can assess your risk of contracting HIV or other sexually transmitted infections. For those suffering from AIDS, the site offers a free discount drug program and lists sources for help. Information also available in Spanish.

| | |
|---|---|
| Name | **HIV Institute** |
| Address | http://hivinsite.ucsf.edu/ |
| Author | Varies with articles and section |
| Contact | info@hivinsite.ucsf.edu |
| Source | University of California San Francisco's (UCSF) AIDS Research Institute, Center for AIDS Prevention Studies, Positive Health Program, Veteran Affairs Medical Center |
| Sponsor | UCSF and several pharmaceutical companies |
| Update | Date given on sections and articles selected |
| Highlights | Comprehensive and current information covering all aspects of HIV and AIDS can be found here. It includes an excellent basic information section that clearly explains how the virus is transmitted and the best ways to prevent the disease. |

| | |
|---|---|
| Name | **National Institute of Diabetes, Digestive, and Kidney Diseases** |
| Address | http://www.niddk.nih.gov/health/digest/digest.htm |
| Author | Professional staff |
| Contact | dkwebmaster@extra.niddk.nih.gov |
| Source | Varies with selection |
| Sponsor | National Institutes of Health |
| Update | Given on articles |
| Highlights | Easy to understand articles and statistics about diseases of the stomach. Links are provided to other sections covering other diseases. Some information is available in Spanish. |

| | |
|---|---|
| Name | **National Institute of Mental Health** |
| Address | http://www.nimh.nih.gov/publicat/index.cfm |
| Author | Varies with article selected |
| Contact | nimhinfo@nih.gov |
| Source | References given on articles |
| Sponsor | National Institutes of Health |
| Update | Given on articles |

Highlights        Contains fact sheets on the symptoms and treatment op-
                  tions on a variety of mental health conditions. It includes
                  a special section on child and adolescent mental health.

Name              **National Kidney Foundation**
Address           http://www.kidney.org
Author            Professional staff
Contact           info@kidney.org
Source            National Kidney Foundation
Sponsor           National Kidney Foundation corporate and other spon-
                  sors are listed on the site
Update            Given on articles
highlights        This site provides an opportunity to learn about kidney
                  disease with an A-to-Z guide. Find out if you qualify for
                  free kidney disease screening offered through the KEEP
                  program. The site also includes information about
                  becoming a kidney donor.

## Prevention Sites

These sites primarily focus on preventive health services such as
screening for illness, immunization, and nutrition. Also included are
sites providing specific information about health interventions that
improve overall health and promote longevity. Don't forget that both
homicide and accidents are leading causes of death and could have
been prevented in many cases. For those with a smoking or weight
problem, the sites listed will provide not only information but also
on-line support to encourage and track the progress made in
improving health. Although not listed, the manufacturer of Nicorette
products and Zyban to aid smoking cessation (GlaxoSmithKline–
www.nicorette.com, www.zyban.com) and the maker of Xenical, a
popular prescription weight loss drug (Roche–www.xenical.com),
also have Web sites. If your doctor suggests any of these medications
for you, visit the sites to learn more about the medication and possible participation in their on-line programs.

*Health Screening Sites*

| | |
|---|---|
| Name | **Clinician's Handbook of Preventive Services, 2nd Edition** |
| Address | http://www.ahcpr.gov/clinic/ppiphand.htm |
| Author | Agency for Health Care Research and Quality |
| Contact | info@ahrq.gov |
| Source | U.S. Preventive Services Task Force and other major authorities |
| Sponsor | Department of Health and Human Services |
| Update | 1998, the third edition is in progress |
| Highlights | Gives recommendations for screening tests, immunizations, and counseling for all age groups and discusses the medical logic behind these recommendations. |

| | |
|---|---|
| Name | **Harvard Center for Cancer Prevention** |
| Address | http://www.yourcancerrisk.harvard.edu |
| Author | Members of the Risk Index Working Group are listed on the site |
| Contact | yourrisk@hsph.harvard.edu |
| Source | Risk Index Working Group of Harvard University |
| Sponsor | Harvard School of Public Health |
| Update | Given on the site |
| Highlights | Estimate your risk for developing any of 12 different types of cancer and learn tips for prevention. This tool works best for people over the age of 40 who have never had cancer. |

| | |
|---|---|
| Name | **The Official U.S. Government Site for People with Medicare** |
| Address | http://www.medicare.gov/health/overview.asp |
| Author | Varies with selection |
| Contact | Contact information available on-site |
| Source | Governmental agencies |
| Sponsor | Department of Health and Human Services |
| Update | Date given on all articles |

Highlights     An excellent resource for finding out what preventative healthcare services are covered benefits under Medicare. In addition, the site gives pointers for finding and selecting a Medicare-covered nursing home. A version of this site is available in Spanish.

*Immunization Sites*

Name          **The National Immunization Program**
Address       http://www.cdc.gov/nip/
Author        Varies with selection
Contact       Multiple contact choices available on the site
Source        Government agencies
Sponsor       Centers for Disease Control
Update        Date given on all articles
Highlights    An excellent site that answers frequently asked questions about immunizations. The most up-to-date immunization schedules are posted here. In addition, programs providing free immunizations for children are listed. A version of this site is available in Spanish.

Name          **National Network for Immunization Information**
Address       http://www.immunizationinfo.org
Author        All articles are physician reviewed
Contact       nnii@idsociety.org
Source        National Network for Immunization Information in partnership with the many medical organizations listed on the site
Sponsor       Annie E. Casey Foundation, Jewish Healthcare Foundation, Robert Wood Johnson Foundation
Update        Dates given on articles
Highlights    Gives the most recent immunization schedules. Provides useful information for parents and health professionals. Discusses in clear language the benefits and risks of commonly recommended shots. Some of the articles are available in Spanish.

| | |
|---|---|
| Name | **Immunization Action Coalition** |
| Address | http://www.immunize.org |
| Author | Varies with article selected |
| Contact | admin@immunize.org |
| Source | Immunization Action Coalition |
| Sponsor | Centers for Disease Control |
| Update | Dates given on articles |
| Highlights | A wealth of information about immunization is presented. In addition, shot requirements by state are available. Gives graphic pictures of people who have contracted diseases that could have been prevented by immunization. |

*Nutrition, Supplements, and Weight Loss Sites*

| | |
|---|---|
| Name | **American Dietetic Association** |
| Address | http://www.eatright.org |
| Author | Varies with selection |
| Contact | Multiple contact choices available on the site |
| Source | Clearly stated, but varies depending upon area of the site you are visiting |
| Sponsor | American Dietetic Association Foundation |
| Update | Date given on all articles |
| Highlights | An excellent site for in-depth food information. Find out about fat, vitamins, minerals, and other components of the food we eat. Get tips and recipes that make it easier to eat five servings of fruit and vegetables daily. Learn about weight loss and dieting from the experts. |

| | |
|---|---|
| Name | **Office of Dietary Supplements** |
| Address | http://dietary-supplements.info.nih.gov |
| Author | Clinical Nutrition Services |
| Contact | ods@nih.gov |
| Source | Governmental agencies |
| Sponsor | National Institutes of Health |
| Update | Date given on articles and fact sheets |

Highlights        Facts sheets available on vitamin and mineral supple-
                  ments. A similar section on botanical supplements is
                  under construction. The site posts warnings on all sup-
                  plements considered to be potentially dangerous to your
                  health.

Name              **Herb Med**
Address           http://www.herbmed.org/index.html
Author            Varies with selection
Contact           research@herbmed.org
Source            Varies with selection
Sponsor           Alternative Medicine Foundation
Update            Dates given on articles
Highlights        This site provides in-depth information about common
                  herbs from folk tradition to an extensive listing of the
                  human clinical data available on individual herbs. In
                  addition, it provides consumer warnings and reports of
                  adverse reactions.

Name              **Consumer Lab.com**
Address           http://www.consumerlab.com
Author            Not applicable
Contact           info@consumerlab.com
Source            Consumer Lab.com's independent laboratory
Sponsor           Consumer Lab.com
Update            Dates of testing given
Highlights        This is an independent laboratory that tests and compares
                  the stated ingredients in differing brands of vitamins,
                  botanicals, and other supplements. To gain full access to
                  their data, a subscription is required. Because regulations
                  for these sorts of products are not standardized, con-
                  sumers of these types of products might want to see brand
                  comparisons and find out what they really are getting.

Name              **Shape Up America**
Address           http://www.shapeup.org

| Author | Information about the editorial board is available on the site |
|---|---|
| Contact | suainfo@shapeup.org |
| Source | Supported by funds from private corporations and foundations that are concerned about weight and physical fitness |
| Sponsor | Shape Up America |
| Update | Update information given on home page |
| Highlights | Includes the Cyber Kitchen where you can get a customized calorie plan, recipes, and other interactive tools designed to promote healthy eating. |

| Name | **Weight Loss and Control** |
|---|---|
| Address | http://www.niddk.nih.gov/health/nutrit/nutrit.htm |
| Author | Primarily governmental agencies |
| Contact | dkwebmaster@extra.niddk.nih.gov |
| Source | National Institute of Diabetes & Digestive & Kidney Diseases |
| Sponsor | National Institutes of Health |
| Update | Date given on articles |
| Highlights | Discusses all aspects of weight control and weight loss including the most common myths associated with dieting. It also has articles targeted at select populations such as teenagers and seniors. |

## Safety Sites

| Name | **National Safety Council** |
|---|---|
| Address | http://www.nsc.org |
| Author | Varies with selection |
| Contact | webmaster@ncs.org |
| Source | Varies with selection |
| Sponsor | National Safety Council, a nongovernment, nonprofit organization established in 1913 to promote safety |
| Update | Given on all articles |
| Highlights | Provides tips that promote safety behind the wheel, at |

work, and at play. This site is filled with startling information. For example, "motor vehicle crashes cause a death every 12 minutes, a disabling injury every 14 seconds."

| | |
|---|---|
| Name | **National Youth Violence Prevention Resource Center** |
| Address | http://www.safeyouth.org |
| Author | Varies with selection |
| Contact | nyvp@safeyouth.org |
| Source | All articles referenced |
| Sponsor | Centers for Disease Control, Federal Working Group on Youth Violence |
| Update | Given on all articles |
| Highlights | This is a good place to find information on prevention and intervention programs on youth violence and suicide. A whole section is devoted to helping parents and guardians recognize youth at risk. |

| | |
|---|---|
| Name | **National Strategy for Suicide Prevention** |
| Address | http://www.mentalhealth.org/suicideprevention/ |
| Author | Varies with selection |
| Contact | ken@mentalhealth.org |
| Source | Varies with selection |
| Sponsor | Multiple governmental agencies |
| Update | Given on articles |
| Highlights | A resource portal to learn about suicide and get prevention advice. This site links to governmental and other sites that deal with the problem of suicide. It features a help number to call if you or a loved one is thinking about suicide. |

## Smoking Cessation Sites

| | |
|---|---|
| Name | **Tobacco Cessation Guideline** |
| Address | http://www.surgeongeneral.gov/tobacco/ |
| Author | Available on article selected |
| Contact | SGWebSite@osophs.dhhs.gov |

Source      Governmental agencies
Sponsor     U.S. Surgeon General
Update      Date given on all articles
Highlights  This site carefully explains the different methods and treatments available to help deal with nicotine addiction. It provides many tips and guidelines for smoking cessation. Much of the information is also available in Spanish.

Name        **American Lung Association**
Address     http://www.lungusa.org/tobacco
Author      Varies with site selected
Contact     Multiple contact choices available on the site
Source      American Lung Association
Sponsor     Volunteers. This is the oldest volunteer health organization in America. The members of their Board of Directors are listed on the site.
Update      Home page updated daily
Highlights  In addition to information why it is healthy to quit smoking, this site offers a 24-hour smoking cessation support program. A version of the site is also available in Spanish.

## Special Interest Sites

These are a group of sites that cater to a specific group of people or deal with a specific treatment or procedure such as medication or surgery. There is overlap with the general information sites, but the specific information you are looking for may be easier to find if you look at a site devoted to a special community. Some of the facts and the resources offered by these sites won't apply to the public at large.

*Age-, Gender-, or Race-Specific Sites*

Name        **Association of Asian Pacific Community Health Organizations**
Address     http://www.aapcho.org

Author        Varies with selection
Contact       webmaster@aapcho.org
Source        Association of Asian Pacific Community Health Orga-
              nizations
Sponsor       Organizations and individual members serving the
              Asian Pacific community
Update        Given on selections
Highlights    Provides brochures in various Asian languages on
              common health problems. Serves as a directory of avail-
              able health services for the Asian community.

Name          **Black Health Online.com**
Address       http://www.blackhealthonline.com/
Author        physicians
Contact       Contact information available on the site
Source        References given on all articles
Sponsor       Black Health Online.com
Update        Given on all articles
Highlights    This site gives basic information about diseases that dis-
              proportionately affect the Black community. In addition
              to basic information about a disease, each article also
              discusses the special impact of the disease on the
              African American population.

Name          **Gay and Lesbian Medical Association**
Address       http://www.glma.org/home.html
Author        Professional staff
Contact       info@glma.org
Source        Gay and Lesbian Medical Association
Sponsor       GlaxoSmithKline, a pharmaceutical company, sponsors
              the current medical information on the site
Update        Dates given on news releases
Highlights    This site provides updates on health concerns facing the
              gay and lesbian community. It provides limited specific
              health information. However, it has a free referral ser-
              vice to healthcare providers across the nation who are
              sensitive to the special needs of this community.

| | |
|---|---|
| Name | **InfoAging.org** |
| Address | http://www.infoaging.org/ |
| Author | Varies with article selected |
| Contact | amfedaging@aol.com |
| Source | Varies with article selected |
| Sponsor | Educational grant from Pfizer |
| Update | Varies with article selected |
| Highlights | This site specializes in issues that face senior citizens and provides an opportunity for feedback. Key articles are accompanied by a survey to find out if the article contained too much or too little medical information. |

| | |
|---|---|
| Name | **National Alliance for Hispanic Health** |
| Address | http://www.hispanichealth.org |
| Author | Professional staff |
| Contact | alliance@hispanichealth.org |
| Source | National Alliance for Hispanic Health |
| Sponsor | Organizations and individuals committed to promoting a strong healthy Hispanic community |
| Update | Dates given on articles |
| Highlights | Basic information is in both English and Spanish and is geared to the Hispanic community. The site lists the 10 most frequent causes of death in Hispanics. It also provides contact information to link to the Hispanic community to resources for help in healthcare matters. |

| | |
|---|---|
| Name | **Kids Health** |
| Address | http://www.kidshealth.org |
| Author | Varies with article selected |
| Contact | Contact information available on the site |
| Source | KidsHealth.org |
| Sponsor | Nemours Foundation |
| Update | Given on articles |
| Highlights | This site is devoted to the medical needs of children. It includes an informative first aid section covering the most common childhood injuries. It also has a special |

health education section designed for children and teenagers.

| | |
|---|---|
| Name | **National Women's Health Center** |
| Address | http://4woman.gov/ |
| Author | Varies with article |
| Contact | Multiple contact options listed on the site |
| Source | Multiple government agencies and organizations |
| Sponsor | Department of Health and Human Services |
| Update | Home page updated daily |
| Highlights | Health topics of particular concern to women prominently featured although information on other diseases is available. The site has a section devoted to current medical news articles focusing on women's issues. A version of this site is available in Spanish. |

| | |
|---|---|
| Name | **New York Online Access to Health–Men's Health** |
| Address | http://www.noah-health.org/english/wellness/healthy living/menshealth.html |
| Author | Varies with selection |
| Contact | noahweb@nyam.org |
| Source | Librarians and specialists in medical education select the sites listed |
| Sponsor | Listed on site and includes the City University of New York, Metropolitan New York Library Council, New York Academy of Medicine, New York Public Library |
| Update | Given on site |
| Highlights | This site is an extensive portal to men's health sites across the Web. The information is organized in a practical and easy-to-use manner. This site is also an excellent resource for general health information. A version of the site is available in Spanish. |

*Drug Information Sites*

| | |
|---|---|
| Name | **Antibiotic Guide** |
| Address | http://hopkins-abxguide.org |

Author       Varies with selection
Contact      abxfeedback@hopkins-abxguide.org.
Source       John Hopkins University Division of Infectious Diseases
Sponsor      Multiple pharmaceutical companies
Update       Date posted on articles
Highlights   Registration is required at no charge to access a wealth of information about antibiotics. You can search by drug or by disease and learn what the experts would prescribe. This site appears more intimidating than it really is. After you click on a topic, a drop-down menu with more familiar medical terms or names of drugs will appear.

Name         **Rx Hope.com**
Address      http://www.rxhope.com/
Author       Specific drug information is from the Physicians Desk Reference (PDR)
Contact      customerservice@rxhope.com
Source       Rx Hope.com
Sponsor      Pharmaceutical and Research Manufacturers of America and participating pharmaceutical companies
Update       Information not given
Highlights   The site provides information about assistance programs that are available for prescription medications. You can search by a partial drug name, by a drug manufacturer name, or choose from a drop-down list. Eligibility requirements are also given.

## Medical Procedure Sites

Name         **Lab Tests Online**
Address      http://www.labtestsonline.org
Author       Professional staff
Contact      labtestsonlin@aacc.org
Source       Laboratory professional
Sponsor      Listed on the site, includes clinical laboratory groups and industry sponsors

Update          Given on each test information page
Highlights      Includes drop-down search boxes by test name or by disease state. In addition to explaining the test and what the results may mean, this site also explains the technique used to obtain the test sample.

Name            **Mediguide.com**
Address         http://www.mediguide.com
Author          Not applicable
Contact         Information available on site
Source          Individual physicians and hospitals
Sponsor         Mediguide.com
Update          Annual renewal required of participating facilities and physicians
Highlights      This site allows you to search by language spoken for a physician or hospital anywhere in the world. The site does not verify the credentials of the physicians listed but depends on information from hospitals where the doctors have privileges. However, when traveling in a foreign country this site could be helpful in finding a doctor you can communicate with.

Name            **Online Specialty Consultations**
Address         https://econsults.partners.org
Author          Not applicable
Contact         Multiple contact sources available on site
Source          Partners Healthcare System, Inc.
Sponsor         Massachusetts General Hospital, Harvard Medical School, Brigham and Women's Hospital, Dana Farber/Partners
Update          Not applicable
Highlights      This site provides on-line second opinions. You and your doctor must be in partnership to use this service. Laws governing the practice of medicine exclude this in seven states so look at the list posted on the site to make sure you live where access to this service is allowed.

| Name | **Your Surgery.com** |
|---|---|
| Address | http://www.yoursurgery.com |
| Author | Physicians specializing in the surgical procedures described |
| Contact | Provided on site |
| Source | Specialty surgeons |
| Sponsor | Your Surgery.com |
| Update | Date given on different sections |
| Highlights | Describes with pictures common surgical procedures. Gives standard pre-operative and post-operative care guidelines. The site educates patients so they will understand a proposed surgical procedure prior to signing the consent form. |

## Sites from Previous Chapters

For your convenience, sites not included above but mentioned in a previous chapter are listed below in order of appearance.

| Reason for citation | Internet address http:// |
|---|---|
| See if your doctor is board certified | www.abms.org |
| See individual state rules regarding the practice of medicine | www.fsmb.org |
| Find out if a doctor has been disciplined | www.docinfo.org |
| Learn about health insurance choices | www.ahcpr.gov/consumer/hlthpln1.htm#choices |
| Evaluate your testosterone level | www.tquiz.com |
| Newborn metabolic testing data | Genes-r-us.uthscsa.edu |
| Learn about air quality | www.aqs.com or www.aerias.com |
| Find out about the river pollution | ga.water.usgs.gov/projects/chatm |

| | |
|---|---|
| Check your child's car seat placement | www.nhtsa.dot.gov |
| Read about Radon | www.epa.gov/iaq/radon |
| Information about Asbestos | www.epa.gov/opptintr/asbestos/help.htm |
| Estimate your risk of breast cancer | bcra.nci.nih.gov/brc/q1htm |
| Blood pressure lowering device | www.resperate.com |
| Find out the latest on bioterrorism | www.cdc.gov |
| Learn safe fish to catch and eat | www.epa.gov/ost/fish |
| Determine your drinking water quality | www.epa.gov/safewater/dwinfo.htm |
| Facts on home water filters | http://www.nsf.org/water.html |
| Be alerted to food recalls | www.fsis.usda.gov/OA/recalls/rec_intr.htm |
| Prepare turkey safely | www.fsis.usda.gov/OA/pubs/tbthaw.htm |
| Be aware of travel precautions | www.cdc.gov/travel |
| Protect your hips | www.safehip.com |
| Estimate your lifespan | www.livingto100.com |
| Obtain a medical identification bracelet | diabetes.org/diabetesforecast/2000BuyersGuide/pg60.htm |
| Estimate your heart attack risk | hin.nhlbi.nih.gov/atpiii/calculator.asp |
| Verify a site's URAC status | websiteaccreditation.urac.org |
| Find out about HonCode | www.hon.ch/Global |
| Read about Internet privacy standards | www.truste.com |
| Use a great search engine | www.google.com |
| Read about new sites | www.fergusonreport.com |

A famous physician of the last century, Sir William Osler, is credited with saying that man is distinguished from other animals by his desire to take medicine. Today perhaps he would say that the desire to find the latest medical information distinguishes modern man from his predecessors. The Internet has brought new meaning to the concept of public health. Medical information isn't just for doctors anymore. Finally it is also readily available to the public. Reliable, current information about even the rarest of medical conditions is now just a mouse click away. Take the time to explore the wealth of medical information available to you on the Internet. As the healthcare consumer, it is in your best health interest to find out all you can. Empower yourself to form a partnership with your doctor for making healthcare decisions. After all, it is your body and your health.

# EMPOWERMENT TIPS

▼ Search the internet for current health information.

▼ Evaluate the quality of all sites you visit.

▼ Check to see if they display the URAC or HonCode seals.

▼ Read privacy policies or look for the Trustmark.

▼ Discuss your findings with your doctor.

# AFTERWORD

There is nothing more important than your health and that of your family. When you are sick, living just isn't as much fun. Yet, we all tend to take good health for granted, especially when we are young. The average lifespan is increasing with every generation. Those born in the 1990s can expect to live well into their seventies. If you want your golden years to be truly golden, now is the time to be proactive about your health. What you do today greatly impacts what you will be capable of doing tomorrow. It is up to you to start living the healthiest lifestyle possible to decrease your risk of serious illness. Of course, no one can predict what will happen and having a healthy lifestyle is not a guarantee for good health. However, the steps necessary to give you the best chance of being a healthy and active senior citizen are easy to take. Why not take them now? Start doing all you can to stave off disease and promote your own health and longevity by exercising regularly, eating five servings of fruit and vegetables daily, and getting a good night's rest.

In addition to living a healthy lifestyle, certain health measures can also help keep you healthy or identify disease early when the chance for cure is the greatest. It is important to keep your immunizations current and be screened for certain diseases on a regular basis. Know what preventive health measures you need and make sure you get them. *Don't leave it up to your doctor to tell you what to do.* Pay attention to your body so you will recognize early symptoms of serious illnesses that might otherwise be overlooked. Be able to report all symptoms to your doctor in a logical and concise manner. Thoroughly discuss and understand all proposed treatment plans. If you aren't sure or feel uncomfortable with a doctor's suggestion, remember you can always get a second opinion. Use the Internet as a source of additional information to be discussed with your doctor. Start treating your doctor as your personal healthcare consultant. It's your body. It's your health. Isn't it time for *you* to be in charge?

. . .

Doctor! Doctor!
I'm watching you;
I'll pay close attention
To what you do.

And as a team,
We'll both decide
The best approach
To  my insides.

Zoe Haugo

# GLOSSARY

## (Say It in English, Please)

To communicate effectively with your doctor or to understand what you are reading on the Internet, you need to speak the language. Doctors are notorious for using big words. Don't be intimidated by the medical lingo. If your doctor uses a word you don't understand, ask for a definition, or at least put a very blank expression on your face. Your doctor knows you don't have a medical background but forgets that the words that play an everyday part of her life may be foreign to you. Don't pretend to understand to be nice or because you are embarrassed. Remember there are no stupid questions, just dumb answers! If you don't let on to your lack of understanding, you're then keeping yourself from using your best health information resource—your doctor.

Use the following glossary as a reference guide. The definitions given aren't meant to be strict dictionary definitions, but rather common usage definitions. In other words, the definitions reflect what most medical personnel mean when they use the word. For example, the *Merriam-Webster Dictionary* defines the word "differential" as "the amount of degree by which things differ." When a doctor talks about a differential, though, he is referring to a test evaluating the white blood cells. It is also possible that the words listed have additional meanings. The definitions below are not comprehensive but are designed to apply to how a term is used in this book. In addition, extra information has been provided to explain the context with which the word is usually used and how it relates to your health or healthcare delivery. Words used in a definition that also have their own glossary entry are set in italics.

**AAFP.** An abbreviation for the American Academy of Family Physicians. Founded in 1947, this organization represents over 93,000 physicians specializing in primary care. This organization was the first to require that its members spend time keeping up-to-date in their field (150 hours of continuing medical education every three years to maintain membership). As a result, many states have adopted similar continuing medical education requirements to maintain licensure to practice medicine.

**AAP.** An abbreviation for the American Academy of Pediatrics. It was founded in 1930 and has about 55,000 members. Their goal is to see that all infants, children, adolescents, and young adults obtain the best healthcare.

**ACOG.** An abbreviation for the American College of Obstetricians and Gynecologists. Founded in 1951, this organization represents over 43,000 physicians specializing in healthcare for women with a focus on prenatal care, pregnancy, and diseases of the female organs.

**ACP-ASIM.** An abbreviation for the American College of Physicians-American Society of Internal Medicine. It is the largest medical specialty society and has about 115,000 members. Members include medical students and physicians in the practice of general internal medicine and its related subspecialties such a cardiology, neurology, nephrology, and oncology.

**Acquired Immunodeficiency Syndrome.** See *AIDS*.

**Acute appointment.** A type of an appointment given at a doctor's office that is reserved for urgent medical problems. This kind of appointment is typically booked no more than forty-eight hours ahead of time.

**Acute Lymphoblastic Leukemia.** A type of *cancer* of the blood in which immature forms of blood cells multiply at the expense of normal cells. It affects more children than adults. *Anemia* and frequent infections are often associated this disease.

**Adult Onset diabetes**. See *Diabetes Mellitus.*

**Adverse reaction.** An unwanted and often unpleasant reaction to a medication that may result in having to stop taking the medication.

**AIDS.** An abbreviation which stands for Acquired Immunodeficiency Syndrome. This disease is caused by the *human immunodeficiency virus (HIV)* and results in damage to the immune system by destroying a certain kind of blood cell known as a helper cell, or T-cell. With loss of protection from the immune system, infected individuals may come down with unusual infections and *cancers* that are often difficult to treat.

**Alanine Transaminase.** See *ALT.*

**Albumin.** A protein in the blood made in the liver that is important in keeping fluid from leaking out from the blood vessels into the tissues of the body. Low levels in the blood can be a sign of liver or kidney disease and/or malnutrition.

**Alkaline Phosphatase (ALP).** An *enzyme* found in all tissues of the body, especially in the liver and bone. With injury or disease, the enzyme is released into the blood. High blood levels may occur with liver disease and/or metastatic bone *cancer.*

**Alpha 1 antitrypsin.** An *enzyme* in the lungs that can be the cause of *chronic obstructive pulmonary disease* if enough isn't available. Treatment with a replacement drug became available after 1990.

**ALT.** An *enzyme* found in many tissues but predominantly in the liver. It is released into the blood with tissue damage or disease. High levels may be seen when liver disease such as *hepatitis* is present.

**Alternative medicine.** An approach to healing and treatment of disease not usually included in medical school curriculums in the United States. This type of medical practice includes herbal medicine, homeopathy, acupuncture, aromatherapy and many others.

**Alzheimer's disease.** A progressive and incurable disease that primarily affects memory. It causes significant disability because affected individuals can lose the ability to care for themselves. It occurs more commonly in the elderly than other age groups. The exact cause is unknown but some genetic risk factors have been identified.

**American Accreditation Healthcare Commission.** A nonprofit organization, also referred to as URAC, that develops standards for the healthcare industry. It currently has a program to accredit healthcare Web sites that meet strict quality standards. Accredited sites may display the URAC seal of approval.

**Anemia.** This is a state in which the ability of the *red blood cells* to supply oxygen to the body is decreased. It may be as a result of blood cell loss, decreased *hemoglobin* in the blood, or decreased volume of the red blood cells. Many different types of anemia exist. Anemia is not really a disease but a sign of another illness or disorder. If the anemia develops gradually, hemoglobin levels can get quite low without symptoms.

**Angina.** A pain or pressure in the chest area usually associated with some type of exertion. It is caused by partially obstructed or blocked flow of blood to the blood vessels of the heart, and is often the first symptom of an impending *heart attack.* It typically is caused by *atherosclerosis,* a build-up of fatty materials in the coronary blood vessels.

**Anthrax.** An infectious disease caused by the spore-forming bacterium *Bacillus anthracis.* Prior to the bombing of the World Trade Center in New York, the disease was contracted primarily by people whose skin came in contact with infected animals or animal products. The disease they usually contracted was cutaneous anthrax. Recently much has been learned about inhalation anthrax, the form of the disease that results from inhalation of spores of the bacterium.

**Antibody.** A protein formed by the body in response to exposure to an *antigen.* Antibodies help the body fight disease.

**Antigen.** A substance capable of making the body create *antibodies* when the immune system recognizes it as a threat.

**Antioxidant.** A substance naturally occurring in fruits and vegetables that is thought to help protect the body on a cellular level from some forms of *cancer* and *atherosclerosis.*

**Anus.** The opening of the bowel to outside the body. Fecal material leaves the body through this opening.

**ApoE4.** A protein in the blood involved with *cholesterol* transport in the body.

**Appeal.** A review of the medical decision-making process involved in a previously denied medical treatment or service in hopes of getting it authorized by a health insurance plan. An appeal may be initiated by the patient, their legal guardian, or their physician. An appeal may also be filed to seek payment from a health insurance company on a previously denied medical claim.

**Arthralgia.** A pain or ache located in a joint of the body such as the knee or hip.

**Asbestos.** A naturally occurring fibrous mineral known to cause *lung cancer.* Since it is heat resistant and has good insulating properties, asbestos has been used extensively in the building industry. Care must be taken when removing asbestos products, so as to prevent the release any of the disease-causing fibers into the air.

**AST (Aspartate Aminotransferase).** An *enzyme* found primarily in the heart, liver, and muscles, AST is usually used with other tests to monitor liver disease. Prior to the ability to test for other more specific enzymes, it was used to help diagnose a *heart attack.*

**Atherosclerosis.** Commonly known as "hardening of the arteries," this condition is the result of *cholesterol*-laden deposits forming in the walls of arteries. These deposits can lead to decreased blood flow or complete blockage of flow through the involved vessel.

**Atrial fibrillation.** A common type of irregular heartbeat marked by rapid activity in the atria, or upper chambers, of the heart. It is an important risk factor for *stroke.*

**Autoimmune disease.** An illness in which the immune system of the body attacks itself. Normally the immune system recognizes itself and does not attack body tissues. However in these disorders, the immune system creates *antibodies* that target normal body cells.

This kind of disease is more common in women. Examples include rheumatoid arthritis, lupus, and Grave's disease.

**Autonomic nervous system.** The part of the nervous system of the body that controls involuntary or automatic functions such as breathing and heartbeat.

**Azotemia.** A high level of nitrogen-containing substances in the blood. The test typically used to discover this condition is a *BUN* level. Azotemia can occur when the kidney aren't working properly.

**Bad cholesterol.** See *LDL cholesterol.*

**Barium enema.** A solution containing barium sulfate is given as an enema to provide the contrast necessary to enhance the visibility of abnormalities during an *X-ray* examination of the colon. This may be used to look for colon *cancer* and other abnormalities.

**Basophil.** A type of *white blood cell* also known as a *granulocyte.* It contains granules that stain with basic dyes.

**Benign Prostatic Hypertrophy.** A noncancerous increase in the size of the *prostate gland.* Typically this occurs with increasing age in men. This condition is sometimes referred to as BPH.

**Bethesda or CIN grading.** A new reporting system giving the results of a *Pap smear* that gives the doctor more meaningful results than the old Class reporting system.

**Bile.** A fluid made in the liver and stored in the gallbladder. It is important in digestion because it helps the body absorb fat.

**Bilirubin.** A breakdown product of *hemoglobin.* When too much bilirubin is accumulated by the body, it leads to jaundice. Bilirubin levels in the blood are useful for the evaluation of liver and gall bladder diseases and other disorders.

**Blood chemistry.** A test that looks at the chemical make up of the blood. Common blood chemistry tests that are ordered look at blood fat levels, blood sugar levels, and blood hormone levels.

**Blood culture.** A test used to identify abnormal organisms in the blood. Blood is withdrawn under sterile conditions and placed on a suitable media and incubated. If growth occurs, the organism is identified.

**Blood pressure.** The pressure against the arterial walls exerted by the blood. Normal adult blood pressure is considered to be a systolic pressure of less than 130 mm of mercury over a diastolic pressure of less than 85 mm of mercury.

**Blood type.** A specific group of blood. Usually refers to type A, B, O, or AB.

**Botulism.** An illness caused by toxins released by the bacterium *Clostridium botulinum* which can cause a fatal paralysis. The disease is usually contracted by eating contaminated food. Recently concern has been raised that this bacterium will be used as a means of bioterrorism.

**BUN (blood urea nitrogen).** A test that measures the level of the substance urea nitrogen in the blood. The test is used primarily to evaluate kidney function.

**Call.** The term used for designating the doctor who is responsible for patient care on holidays and after normal office hours. The doctor is "on call" and must be available for patient duties. A "call schedule" will list which doctor is responsible on any given day.

**Cancer.** An uncontrolled and unnecessary growth of cells within the body. The cancer cells can invade healthy tissues locally and may spread to other parts of the body. Cancer is the second leading cause of death in the United States. The most common adult cancers are lung, colon, breast, and prostate.

**Cancer grade.** A way of stating how malignant a cancer is. Cancer cells that hardly resemble normal tissue are thought to grow faster and spread more easily. Many cancers are graded I to IV with grade IV being the worst kind of cells.

**Cancer stage.** This refers to how much the initial cancer has spread to the rest of the body. Staging indicates if the cancer is still contained within an organ or has escaped and invaded surrounding tissues and/or formed new cancers elsewhere in the body. Usually cancers are staged I to IV with stage IV being the worst.

**Cardiovascular disease.** Any disease that affects the heart or the arteries and veins. This includes disease of the blood vessels caused by *atherosclerosis* or hardening of the arteries and other diseases such those that affect the heart muscle.

**CBC.** See *complete blood count.*

**Central nervous system.** The brain, spinal cord, and cranial nerves. It does not include the peripheral nerves.

**Chancre.** The first sign of the sexually transmitted infection *syphilis*. A painless ulcer usually occurs somewhere on the genitalia but it can be located elsewhere on the body. Left alone, it will disappear but the disease is still present and may continue to cause harm if not treated.

**Chlamydia.** This generally refers to the sexually transmitted infection caused by the bacterium *Chlamydia trachomatis*. It is the most common sexually transmitted disease in the United States. When the infection is not recognized early and treated, it may cause infertility. The use of condoms during sexual activity helps prevent the spread of this disease.

**Chloride.** One of the negative ions in the blood that contribute to many body functions. It was the first *electrolyte* to be routinely measured in the blood. Chloride levels tend to shift in the same direction as sodium levels. High levels may be seen with dehydration and low levels with prolonged vomiting.

**Cholesterol.** A waxy substance present in foods of animal origin, in the body cholesterol is made by the liver. High levels are associated with an increased risk of *heart attack* and *stroke*. It is important to know your levels of both high density or good cholesterol and low density or bad cholesterol. Eating a diet containing no more than 30 percent of calories from fat is one method used to help prevent development of high blood cholesterol levels.

**Chronic bronchitis.** The presence of a cough producing sputum for at least three consecutive months. The condition is the result of an inflammation of the bronchi of the lungs. It is most commonly caused by smoking.

**Chronic Obstructive Pulmonary Disease.** An incurable disease of the lungs that results in progressive debilitation. The lung loses its normal elasticity, air sacs become enlarged, and it becomes increasingly difficult to move air in and out the lungs. The disease is usually attributed to the presence of *chronic bronchitis* and *emphysema*. Smoking is the biggest risk factor for this major cause of death.

**Claudication.** A discomfort or pain in the lower leg caused by exercise and relieved by rest. It is the result of the leg muscles not getting enough oxygen. It is a symptom of vascular disease and may be caused by *cholesterol* deposits blocking the flow of blood in the main arteries of the leg.

**Claustrophobia.** A fear of being in any enclosed space such as an elevator.

**Colon.** The large intestine. It is divided into the ascending, the transverse, the descending, and sigmoid colon. The large intestine helps in the digestive process and in the formation, storing, and passage of stool. *Cancer* of the colon is the second most common cancer in the United States.

**Colorectal cancer.** A *cancer* located in the large intestine or rectum. It occurs primarily in people over age fifty. Early screening and diagnosis have been proven to lower the death rate from this common cancer. Screening should be done on an annual basis with the fecal occult blood test or less frequently with other screening tests such as colonoscopy. Initial symptoms of the disease may be vague but usually include some change in bowel habits.

**Colposcopy.** An examination of the vaginal walls and cervix with a culposcope. This instrument is lighted and provides magnification to help detect the presence of abnormal cells. At the time of the examination, biopsies can be taken. Colposcopy is usually preformed to get more precise information about abnormalities found on a *Pap smear*.

**Complementary medicine.** Methods to promote health that are outside of the scope of the traditional Western practice of medicine. Some of these methods have been proven to be effective and often complement traditional Western medical practice.

**Complete blood count.** A test to determine the number of *red blood cells, white blood cells, hemoglobin,* and *platelets* present in the blood. It is a commonly ordered test used to evaluate any condition that might affect the make up of the blood.

**Computed tomography.** A method of picture taking where *X-rays* are sent from more than one direction at the body. Tomography machines are now capable of reconstructing more than just cross sectional or axial images of parts of the human body. Thus the term CAT (computed axial tomography) scan is no longer appropriate. Because the tomography images or slices can be stacked upon each other to create a three-dimensional model of what is being examined, CTs are better than regular X-ray to show the relationship of structures. Ultra fast CT also known as *electron beam tomography* is accomplished by rotating the X-ray beam at targets placed around the patient rather than moving the patient through the scanner. This is especially good for looking at the structure of blood vessels. Studies are underway evaluating this technique for predicting *heart attacks* based on the amount of calcium visualized in the coronary blood vessel walls.

**Congenital anomaly.** A malformation or defect that occurs while the baby is inside the womb. It is present at birth.

**Congenital hypothyroidism.** An inadequate level of thyroid hormone in the baby's body at the time of birth. If not corrected promptly, this can lead to severe mental retardation known as cretinism.

**Connective tissue.** The tissue in the body that provides support or connects to other parts. Examples include bone, tendons, and cartilage.

**Consent form.** The form signed by a patient or a patient's legal guardian giving permission for a healthcare provider to perform a procedure or provide a treatment. By signing the form, the patient acknowledges that he is aware of what is going to be done and is aware of all of the possible outcomes and thus is an informed patient.

**Contagious.** The period of time during an illness when on person is capable of giving or spreading a disease to another individual.

**Contrast.** A substance that is used to increase the visibility of a structure during an *X-ray* or other imaging procedure. Usually contrast material is swallowed, injected into a blood vessel, or given as an enema.

**Co-payment.** The out-of-pocket money paid by a person with health insurance when he receives care from a healthcare facility or fills a prescription. This fee is in addition to the healthcare insurance premium. Co-payments were designed to keep premiums for basic health coverage more affordable to the general public.

**COPD.** See *chronic obstructive pulmonary disease.*

**Creatinine.** This substance is a breakdown product from the muscles excreted by the kidneys. As muscle mass does not change rapidly, a high level in the blood usually means that the kidneys are not working properly.

**Creutzfeldt-Jakob disease.** A fatal *dementia* thought possibly to be caused by an agent related to a *central nervous system* disease found in cattle. It causes a rapidly progressive dementia accompanied by muscle jerking and difficulty walking.

**Cytoplasm.** All of the material inside an individual cell except the nucleus.

**DEET.** The chemical substance n-diethyl-3-methylbenzamide. It is used in many popular insect repellants.

**Dementia.** An incapacitating loss of mental function. Most cases are progressive and irreversible. In the elderly, *Alzheimer's disease* is the most frequent type.

**Dental history.** A part of a person's past medical history that focuses on oral health. It includes frequency of evaluations and the various dental treatments received. In evaluating many medical conditions, the dental history gives the doctor valuable clues. For example, people who wore braces are more likely to suffer from jaw pain known as temporal mandibular joint syndrome (TMJ).

**Diabetes.** This condition, properly known as Diabetes Mellitus, results from failure of the pancreas to produce enough *insulin* or from the tissues of the body becoming resistant to the action of insulin. As a result, the sugar or glucose levels in the blood become abnormally elevated. Diabetes that is the result of insulin resistance is known as Non-Insulin Dependant Diabetes Mellitus (*NIDDM*). This type of diabetes usually occurs in adults. Diabetes that is caused by the pancreas not producing enough insulin is known as Insulin Dependent Diabetes Mellitis (*IDDM*). This kind of diabetes typically occurs in young people. *Gestational diabetes* is a form of diabetes that occurs while a woman is pregnant. It is associated with a higher than normal risk of developing NIDDM later in life. The treatment of NIDDM usually does not include insulin injections. Lifestyle changes, such as a diabetic diet, weight control, and regular exercise, are utilized along with oral sugar lowering agents to gain sugar control. In severe cases, insulin injections may be needed instead of oral agents. IDDM requires insulin to maintain control of blood sugar levels. Control of the blood sugar is necessary to help prevent macrovascular complications, such as a *heart attack*, and microvascular complications, such as blindness, from the disease.

**Diarrhea**. The frequent passage of watery and unformed stools. Often the stooling is associated with abdominal cramps and gas. Severe diarrhea can serious health problems such as dehydration and *electrolyte* imbalances.

**Diastolic blood pressure.** The pressure of the blood when the ventricles of the heart are filling with blood. Diastolic pressures of greater than 85 are considered high.

**Differential diagnosis.** A listing of possible diseases a patient might have based on the symptoms of an illnesses, the physical examination, and results of any testing or procedures that have been performed. Each of the diseases will differ from the others in a way that will allow a doctor, with additional information or testing, to determine a final diagnosis.

**DNA.** An abbreviation for deoxyribonucleic acid, a molecule that carries genetic information in humans. It is found in chromosomes and consists of two long chains that twist around each other to form a double helix. The first evidence that DNA carried genetic material was discovered in 1944. In 1962 James Watson and Francis Crick won a Nobel Prize for figuring out the helical pattern of DNA.

**Domain**. A term for the ending of a Web site address. Top level domains are the most common endings and are readily recognized by Web surfers. New top level domains are being created, but the current ones include ".gov," ".org," ".edu," ".com," and ".net."

**Drug interaction.** The effect one drug has on another when taken together. The result may be good or bad. It is important for healthcare consumers to be aware that interactions occur and to let their doctor know all medications that are taken, including over-the-counter preparations and herbs or supplements. The chances of having a bad interaction increase markedly with the number of drugs taken.

**Ductal breast cancer.** A cancer that starts in the ducts of the breast. In the early stages a breast mass isn't able to be felt with this kind of cancer. Mammograms are good at detecting this cancer while it is still in an early stage.

**Dumping.** A practice of transferring difficult patients or those without health insurance to another provider or healthcare facility for evaluation and treatment.

**EBCT**. See *electron beam computed tomography*.

**Electrocardiogram (EKG).** A graph of the electrical activity of the heart. It consists of a tracing of waves created by the contraction of the atria and ventricles moving blood through the heart. It is used to help in the diagnosis of irregular heart beats, *heart attacks*, and other conditions that affect the heart. The electrocardiogram is frequently referred to as an EKG or ECG.

**Electrolytes.** Various chemicals that can carry an electrical charge. In the blood they exist as acids, bases, and salts. When a test for serum electrolytes is ordered, typically *sodium*, chloride, *potassium*, and calcium levels are obtained. Doctors get very concerned when potassium levels are abnormal because this can lead to fatal irregular heart rhythms. Electrolyte levels can also be ordered on a stool sample to help evaluate the cause of a persistent diarrhea.

**Electron beam computed tomography**. A newer type of imaging also known as ultra fast computed tomography. It is accomplished by rotating the *X-ray* beam at targets placed around the patient rather than moving the patient through the scanner. This is especially good for looking at the structure of blood vessels. Studies are underway to evaluate this technique for predicting *heart attacks* based on the amount of calcium visualized in the coronary blood vessel walls.

**Emphysema.** A chronic and progressive lung disease marked by an abnormal increase in the size of the air sacs and the development of scar tissue. As the disease progresses, it becomes increasingly more difficult to breathe. Since there is no cure for this disease, prevention is critical. The best was to prevent this disease is to never start smoking and to avoid second-hand smoke whenever possible. A small number of people will develop emphysema because they have inherited an *alpha-1-antitrypsin* deficiency.

**Encounter form.** The form the doctor or mid-level provider hands you upon completion of your office visit. The type of office visit you are being charged for, tests and procedures that occurred, any supplies used, and your diagnosis usually are noted on this sheet. You should review this form as you would the check at a restaurant.

**Environmental Protection Agency.** This is a governmental agency whose mission is to protect human health and to safeguard the environment. The head of this agency, frequently referred to as the EPA, is appointed by the president of the United States.

**Enzyme.** A protein that changes the rate of a chemical reaction without being changed itself. Diseases can be caused by lack of enzymes.

**Eosinophil.** A type of *white blood cell* known as a *granulocyte*. The coarse granules within the cell can be stained with acids. Eosinophils are important in allergic reactions and serum blood levels of eosinophils often rise with allergies.

**EPA.** See *Environmental Protection Agency.*

**Epstein-Barr virus.** Associated with the disease mononucleosis or "mono," infection with the Epstein-Barr virus usually causes a transient and minor fatigue and general tiredness but the infection can be much more serious in people with a poorly functioning immune system as those with *AIDS*. In the past, the Epstein-Barr virus was thought to be a cause of chronic fatigue syndrome but this has been disproven.

**Erythrocyte.** A mature *red blood cell*. Red blood cells (RBCs), are formed in the bone marrow and are used by the blood to carry oxygen. For this reason, people who live in high altitudes where the air is thin tend to have higher levels than usual. People unaccustomed to a high altitude areas may experience unexpected shortness of breath with activities until their body produces more red blood cells.

**Erythrocyte sedimentation rate (ESR).** A blood test that measures the rate *red blood cells* settle in a tube over time. This test is a nonspecific test that measures the presence of inflammation. It is often used to monitor treatment or reoccurrence of a disease once a diagnosis has been established. If you have a mild vague complaint that your doctor can't really pinpoint, and the doctor feels no further testing is necessary, a normal sedimentation rate will reassure you and your doctor that nothing too serious is probably going on. This test may also be referred to as an ESR or a sed rate.

**Estrogen.** The female sex hormone produced by the ovary, estrogen is a key ingredient in birth control pills. In addition, it is given after menopause to women desiring hormonal replacement therapy. Certain *cancers* are sensitive to the actions of this hormone.

**False positive.** A test result that is erroneously positive for a condition when that condition is in actuality not present. For example, a screening test for the sexually transmitted infection *syphilis* may be positive for other reasons when the disease is not present.

**Family history.** A part of the medical history focusing on the health of the patient's blood relatives. It is of interest to the doctor because many illnesses run in families. The empowered healthcare consumer will ask a doctor about preventative measures that may stave off diseases known to run in his family.

**Family physician.** A physician who is trained in the medical specialty of family practice. Family physicians provide preventative services and continuing comprehensive medical care to each member of a family regardless of sex, age, or type of problem. They are skilled advocates for the patient in all health-related matters.

**Family practice.** The medical specialty which provides healthcare for individuals and families. The scope of family practice covers all ages, both sexes, and all diseases.

**Fasting.** A state of not having eaten any food for a set period of time. Before a blood test that needs to drawn in the fasting state, patients are usually requested not to eat after midnight and to come in for the test the first thing in the morning or advised to go nine hours without food.

**Fecal–oral transmission.** A common method for passing infection for one person to another. Germs in the stool are inadvertently transferred to another individual who then may unknowingly inoculate himself with the germ. Door knobs and other handles are big culprits in this kind of transmission.

**Fever.** An elevation in normal body temperature. Oral temperatures range from about 97.6° to 99.6°F. Normal temperatures vary depending upon the time of day, with the lowest readings occur in the early morning. In practice, an adult is not felt to have a significant fever unless it is greater than 100.4°F. Fever is part of the body's own way of fighting disease. Higher body temperatures may contribute to the death of disease-producing organisms. Fevers of 104°F or higher, however, can be harmful, especially to children, so a doctor should be contacted immediately and fever-lowering measures should be instituted.

**First degree relative.** A blood relative who is no more than one generation removed. For example, your mother or your sister is a first degree relative.

**Follow-up appointment.** An appointment you make with a health-care provider to review the status of your health or condition. These kinds of appointments usually take less time than an initial visit because a diagnosis has already been established.

**Food recall**. A voluntary action by a company to remove unsafe products from market shelves.

**Formulary**. A listing of drugs that will be paid for under the pharmacy benefits rules by a health insurance plan when prescribed for a certain condition. Most formularies contain both brand name and generic medications depending upon the condition being treated and the therapeutic options that are available.

**Free PSA.** The unbound prostate specific antigen circulating in the blood. The diagnosis of *prostate cancer* is suggested when the levels of free PSA in the blood are less than 25 percent of total prostate specific antigen levels.

**Gamma Glutamyl Transferase.** An *enzyme* found in the liver, bile ducts, and kidney. It is used in combination with other tests to evaluate disease in this area of the body. This enzyme is frequently high in people who abuse alcohol. This test is also called a GGT.

**Gangrene.** The death of tissue. Usually this is the result of poor or absent blood supply to an area of the body. It generally refers to an infection resulting from the gas-producing bacteria *Clostridium.*

**General practice.** A broad term used to describe the practice of physicians who have not completed a medical specialty residency training program.

**Genetics.** The study of heredity. Your genes determine to some degree your susceptibility to certain diseases. However just because everyone in your family has come down with an illness does not mean that you will. Genetic research has taught us a lot about identification of risks and prevention.

**Gestational diabetes.** A type of diabetes which develops during pregnancy. It usually goes away after delivery of the baby but may recur later in life. It is important to treat gestational diabetes to prevent abnormalities in the baby and complications in the mother.

**Gingivitis.** An inflammation or infection of the gums in the mouth. It is characterized by redness, swelling, and gums that bleed easily. Gum disease is a leading cause of tooth loss in adults. Good oral hygiene, regular brushing and flossing of the teeth, will prevent gingivitis.

**GGT.** See *Gamma Glutamyl Transferase.*

**Glomerulonephritis.** A type of kidney disease caused by inflammation of an internal part of the kidney known as glomeruli. This impairs the kidney's ability to filter the blood. Consequently protein is spilled into the urine. It frequently follows infections of the upper respiratory tract caused by certain strains of the *streptococci* bacteria, but can also be caused by other diseases. This condition may be temporary or progress to chronic nephritis and ultimately kidney failure.

**Glucose.**  A simple sugar that results from carbohydrate metabolism. It is a source of energy for most cells. Higher than normal blood levels of glucose is one of the main signs of the disease *diabetes*.

**Glycalated Hemoglobin**.  A type of *hemoglobin* that has glucose bound to it. The amount of *glucose* that gets bound is related to the average amount of glucose in the blood over time. A glycalated hemoglobin level, also known as a Hemoglobin $A_{1c}$, reflects how well a diabetic patient has controlled his blood sugar over the last several months. It is a test that may to be performed without fasting. High levels tell the doctor that the patient is not taking the best care of himself.

**Goiter.**  An enlargement of the thyroid gland which may be caused by inflammation, iodine deficiency, *cancer*, or any condition that results in abnormal thyroid function.

**Gonorrhea.**  A sexually transmitted infection caused by the bacterium *Neisseria gonnorrhoeae*. It causes inflammation of the reproductive tract and organs. Most men will notice a discharge from their penis but many women will not experience symptoms. Untreated, the disease can result in infertility. The use of a condom helps prevent transmission of this disease. The incidence of gonorrhea has recently started to rise in the United States after several years of steady decline, so make sure you practice safe sex.

**Good cholesterol**.  See *HDL cholesterol*.

**Granulocyte.**  A type of *white blood cell*. Included in this group are *neutrophils, eosinophils,* and *basophils*.

**Grave's disease.**  A specific type of thyroid disease. It causes the thyroid to produce too much thyroid hormone. As a result, the gland may enlarge and the eyes may appear to be popping out of the head. Symptoms may include nervousness, weight loss, and hair loss.

**Gynecologist.**  A physician who specializes in diseases that affect the reproductive organs of women.

***H. Pylori.***  A bacteria, *helicobacter pylori*, that has been found to cause peptic ulcers. It can be treated with a combination of antibiotics.

Diagnosis is available by several different methods including a blood test, a breath test, and bacterial culture.

**HbA1c.** See *Glycalated hemoglobin.*

**HDL cholesterol.** The good cholesterol. Increased levels of high density lipoproteins (HDL) are felt to be protective against heart disease. A good level of this kind of cholesterol is greater than 35 mg/dl.

**Health maintenance organization.** A prepaid health plan that provides comprehensive medical care. Although healthcare coverage is usually very good with these plans, the choice of healthcare providers and facilities that can be used may be limited.

**Health on the Net Foundation.** This is a nonprofit international organization that provides leadership in setting standards for health Web sites. Its mission is to help people find reliable medical information on-line. To that end they have developed the *HonCode* seal which only qualified sites may display.

**Health plan.** An organization that provides health insurance. With any plan there will be a basic premium that you have to pay to be eligible for the health insurance coverage and additional fees such as deductibles and *co-payments* for certain services.

**Heart attack.** A blockage of a coronary blood vessel resulting in loss or damage to heart muscle. The blockage prevents oxygen from getting to an area of the heart. If blood supply is not restored within a few hours, the heart muscle dies. If you experience symptoms that are suggestive of a heart attack, call 911 immediately and take an aspirin. In addition to reducing inflammation, aspirin thins the blood and may allow some blood to get through the blocked area.

***Helicobacter pylori.*** See *H. pylori.*

**Hematocrit.** The volume of packed *red blood cells* in a given volume of blood. This test is sometimes referred to as a packed cell volume. It is often used to monitor blood loss or to detect the *anemia.*

**Hematology test.** A test that looks at the components that make up the blood itself, not the other chemicals that are carried by the blood. Typically these are tests that look at the *white blood cells*, the *red blood cells*, or the *platelets.*

**Hemoglobin A$_{1c}$.** See *Glycalated hemoglobin.*

**Hemoglobinopathy.** Any one of a group of blood disorders that are associated with abnormal forms of *hemoglobin* in the blood. Usually these diseases are inherited.

**Hepatitis.** An inflammation of the liver. Usually it is caused by an infection, but alcohol, other toxic chemicals, and drugs may also cause hepatitis. *Immunization* is available to protect against certain forms of this disease. Depending upon the type of hepatitis contracted, the disease may be mild and short-lived or much more serious. Heavy alcohol drinkers should avoid taking acetaminophen (Tylenol) to prevent a hangover after binging since the combination can result in severe damage to the liver.

**Hepatitis A.** An infection of the liver caused by the Hepatitis A virus. This is the kind of hepatitis you get from contact with contaminated food and water or contact with an infected individual. Symptoms of the disease are similar to the flu but include jaundice.

**Hepatitis B.** An infection of the liver caused by the Hepatitis B virus. It is transmitted by blood and other body fluids. Some of the ways you can contract the disease are by sharing needles, having your body pierced with contaminated equipment, or by having unsafe sex. Hepatitis B may become chronic hepatitis and eventually lead to liver failure and death.

**Hepatitis C.** An infection of the liver caused by the Hepatitis C virus. It is caused by coming in contact with infected blood or body fluids. The majority of patients who get this infection develop chronic hepatitis. The disease can be prevented by taking the same precautions recommended to prevent Hepatitis B.

**Herd immunity.** The effect of immunizing large groups of people. Because the immunized people can't catch a disease, it is harder for that disease to spread within a community.

**Hereditary disease.** A disease that you may contract because of the genes you inherited from your parents.

**Herpes.** A viral disease that causes small blisters around the mouth or genitalia or on other parts of the body. Although different forms of the disease exist, when using just the word "herpes" most are referring to genital herpes, a sexually transmitted infection that you have for life. There is no cure for the disease but the number of outbreaks tends to lessen over time. Medicine is available to reduce the severity of attacks and prevent outbreaks. However, you still can be contagious even when skin lesions aren't present.

**Hi-Ethics.** This is a nonprofit organization that established a set of fourteen principles to guide the development of healthcare Web sites. These principles are the basis for the URAC accreditation program insuring quality of health information Web sites.

**Hippocrates.** The Greek physician (460–375 B.C.E.) credited with being the Father of Medicine. He developed ethical standards for the practice of medicine called the Hippocratic Oath. At one time, medical students were required to take this oath prior to graduation from medical school.

**History of present illness.** A complete description of the current medical symptoms given by the patient to the doctor. It is important to be completely honest and as specific as possible.

**HIV.** An abbreviation for a serious disease-causing virus called the human immunodeficiency virus. Infection with this virus causes a loss of the immune function of the body and the development of *Acquired Immunodeficiency Syndrome (AIDS)*. Although newer medicines have slowed the progression of the disease to full-blown AIDS, there is still no cure for this infection.

**Hodgkin's disease.** A specific type of *cancer* known as a *lymphoma* that involves the lymph tissues. It is more common in young adults. The presence of a big lymph node or mass without a known cause such as a sore throat or other infection can lead to the diagnosis of this cancer.

**HonCode.** A set of eight ethical principles of management for Web developers of health-related sites. These principles were developed by the *Health on the Net Foundation* to promote reliable and trustworthy medical information on the Web.

**Hormone receptors.** A structure in a cell that can combine with a hormone to change the function of the cell. The hormone receptor assay test is important in breast *cancer* to determine if the cancer can be treated or influenced by hormones.

**Human Immunodeficiency Virus.** See *HIV.*

**Hyperplasia.** An excessive growth of normal cells in the normal cellular arrangement for an organ. Because the tissue growth doesn't consist of abnormal cells, this isn't considered cancerous.

**Hypertension.** Having higher than normal *blood pressure.* In adults levels above 130/85 are considered high. Uncontrolled high blood pressure puts you at risk for having a *heart attack* or *stroke.* Simple things like regular exercise and watching the amount of salt in your diet can help prevent hypertension.

**Hyperthyroidism.** A condition in which one has too much thyroid hormone in the body. There are many causes for this condition but the most common is caused by *Grave's disease.* Symptoms are multiple and may include nervousness, insomnia, weight loss, and palpitations of the heart.

**IDDM.** An abbreviation for the disease Insulin Dependant *Diabetes* Mellitus. This is the type of diabetes that usually affects younger individuals and was once called juvenile onset diabetes. It is primarily caused by an inability of the pancreas to produce enough *insulin.* Treatment requires the use of insulin and following a diabetic diet.

**Immunization.** The use of vaccination or the injection of immune globulins to keep individuals from getting a disease. Small doses of an *antigen* are introduced into the body so that the immune system will learn how to attack and defend the body against certain diseases without inducing illness. Four types of vaccines are currently used to create this action by the immune system. A vaccine may be made from a weakened live virus, from a dead virus, from a toxin produced by the virus, or from a synthetic or bioengineered substance that will trigger the immune response.

**Impotence.** The inability of a man to achieve or maintain an erection capable of sexual intercourse. Impotence can be an early sign of *diabetes* and/or heart disease. Treatment is available so men having this problem are encouraged to discuss it with their doctor.

**Incontinence.** Loss of control over when you go to the bathroom. This term usually is used in regard to loss of control of your urine but also applies to loss of control of your stool. Medicine is available to control what is being termed "overactive" bladder. In addition, many discrete absorbent products are available that can be worn to prevent soiling of clothing. (Products are available in different sizes and separate styles designed for either men or women.)

**Insulin.** A hormone made by the pancreas necessary for the metabolism of sugar in the body. As a drug, it is used to treat the disease *diabetes*.

**Insurance card.** A card which shows what kind of health insurance you have. The card will have your group number and brief description of your covered benefits and required *co-payments*. Typically the back of the card tells you what procedures require pre-certification by the insurance company and how to contact them.

**Internist.** A doctor who specializes in the practice of internal medicine. This specialty is limited to the overall health and well being of adults.

**Ischemia.** A temporary inadequate flow of blood to an area of the body, ischemia usually causes pain. *Angina*, the chest pain associated with heart disease, is a form of ischemia.

**Juvenile onset diabetes.** See *IDDM*.

**LDL cholesterol.** The bad *cholesterol*. Most cholesterol is carried by lipoproteins in the blood. Low density lipoprotein or LDL seems to carry cholesterol to various tissues in the body. Consequently it is the kind of cholesterol that is associated with the formation of plaques in the blood vessels. Currently individuals with a history of heart disease are recommended are keep their LDL cholesterol level down to less than 100 mg/dl. With no history of heart disease, a level of less than 130 mg/dl currently is considered acceptable.

**Leukemia.** A type of *cancer* that affects the blood. Normal blood cells are replaced with immature ones. As the number of normal cells decrease, *anemia*, infection, and bleeding often start occurring.

**Leukocyte.** A *white blood cell* (WBC). There are two kinds, *granulocytes* and agranulocytes. The granulocytes contain large granules that can be stained different colors and visualized under a microscope. These are sometimes also referred to as polymorphonuclear or polys because they have a nucleus with several parts. The granulocytes are the *eosinophils*, the *basophils*, and the *neutrophils*. Agranulocytes don't contain the granules. These are the *lymphocytes* and the *monocytes*. Leukocytes are part of the immune system and help the body fight disease.

**Leukocyte count.** A test which counts the number and kind of *leukocytes* present in the blood.

**Life event.** Any happening, good or bad, that affects your life. Marriages, divorces, and births of children are all considered major life events.

**Lipoprotein.** A chemical in the blood bound to fat. LDL and HDL are the most important lipoproteins in the body in terms of predicting the risk for heart disease and *stroke*.

**Lobe.** A fairly well defined part of an organ.

**Lobular breast cancer.** A breast *cancer* that originates in the lobes of breast tissue. With this kind of cancer, a woman may find a lump when she performs a self breast exam.

**Lobule.** A smaller part of a lobe of the breast. The lobules become the bulbs and produce breast milk. The lobules are surrounded by tiny ducts which connect to the nipple.

**Lung cancer.** The most deadly form of *cancer* in the United States. It is associated with smoking. Most people die within five years of being diagnosed with this disease. There currently is no recommended screening test for this cancer in people without symptoms. A chest *X-ray* is a diagnostic test used to find the cancer in people with symptoms.

**Lymphocyte.** A type of *white blood cell* known as an agranulocyte. Lymphocytes in the blood may increase when you have a viral infection.

**Lymphoma.** A *cancer* the affects the lymph tissues. They are classified as *Hodgkin's disease* and *non-Hodgkin's lymphomas*. Typically non-Hodgkin's lymphoma occurs in older people while Hodgkin's affects young adults.

**Macrovascular.** Having to do with the bigger blood vessels of the body. Macrovascular complications of diabetes include heart attacks and strokes

**Mad Cow Disease.** An illness that affects the *central nervous system* of cows. It is transmissible but the causative agent is not fully known. There is believed to be an association with the human disease which causes a fatal *dementia, Creutzfeldt-Jakob disease.* The fear is that eating meat from an infected cow will produce dementia of this type in humans. Mad Cow disease is primarily a problem in England and has not yet been found in cows in the United States.

**Magnetic resonance imaging.** An imaging technique that uses magnetic fields and radio waves rather than *X-rays* to produce an image. Often called an MRI, the imaging can be performed through clothing but metal objects may not be worn. People with pacemakers or metal plates should alert their doctor. This form of imaging can detect subtle differences in various body tissues.

**Mammogram.** An *X-ray* examination of the breast tissue. When taken with digital film, the radiologist can rotate and enhance the images and sometimes prevent the need for additional pictures to be taken. To get the best mammogram go to a federally accredited center.

**Medical emergency.** A condition of such severity that failure to get immediate medical attention could reasonably be expected to result in serious impairment to bodily functions or loss of life. The clause "reasonably expected" or "perceived by the patient" is usually included in the definition of an emergency to protect healthcare consumers from managed healthcare plans refusing to pay emergency room charges in certain situations.

**Meningitis.** An infection or inflammation on the lining of the brain and spinal cord. It is a serious condition that may result in permanent brain damage. Typical symptoms include with a high fever and a headache. The disease can worsen very rapidly, so if meningitis is suspected, seek medical attention immediately. *Immunization* is available against certain types of meningitis.

**Menopause.** The period in a woman's life when she permanently stops having menstrual periods. Most women stop menstruating in their late forties and early fifties. Women who smoke tend to go through menopause earlier than nonsmokers.

**Metastatis.** A spread of *cancer* from one part of the body to another.

For example, the cancer may spread by being transported through the blood stream or by entering the lymph system.

**MI (myocardial infarction).** See *heart attack.*

**Microvascular.** Having to do with the small blood vessels of the body. Diabetics often develop a microvascular complication of their disease such as blindness, kidney failure, and loss of sensation to the feet.

**Monocyte.** A type of *white blood cell* known as an agranulocyte. Monocytes have a single nucleus as opposed to the polymorphonuclear *leukocytes.* Monocytes can take in or consume foreign material to help the body fight disease.

**Mononucleosis.** An infectious disease caused by the *Epstein-Barr virus.* It is common in young adults and is frequently referred to as the "kissing disease" because the virus can be transmitted by salvia. Fatigue, sore throat, and fever are the main symptoms of the disease.

**Monounsaturated.** A term used to describe a type of fat. In chemistry fats are compounds composed of fatty acids. When the fatty acid contains one double bond between carbon atoms, it is monounsaturated. This is the type of fat found in oils that are felt to be healthier eating choices such as olive or canola oil.

**Mortality rate.** A death rate. In the United States the top causes of mortality are heart disease, *cancer, stroke, Chronic Obstructive Pulmonary Disease,* and accidents.

**Myocardial infarction (MI).** See *heart attack.*

**National Highway Traffic Safety Administration.** A division of the U.S. Department of Transportation which attempts to reduce deaths and injuries from motor vehicle accidents by setting and enforcing safety performance standards.

**Neonatal period.** The first thirty days of a newborn's life. It is the most critical period in a baby's life.

**Neuroblastoma.** A type of *cancer* that occurs primarily in infants and children. It develops from the tissues that form the sympathetic nervous system. An unusual abdominal mass in a child may alert parents to this tumor.

**Neurofibrillary tangles.** A finding in the brain cells that is associated with the *dementia*-causing illness known as *Alzheimer's disease.*

**Neurtic plaques.** A microscopic finding in the brain cells associated with *Alzheimer's disease.*

**Neutrophil.** The most common type of *white blood cell.* Neutrophils are critical in helping the body fight infection. They tend to increase with infections caused by bacteria. Neutrophils contain large granules that stain and a nucleus with multiple lobes and so are also called granulocytes and polymorphonuclear *leukocytes.*

**NIDDM.** An abbreviation for Non-Insulin Dependent Diabetes Mellitus. It is caused by an increased resistance of the body to the presence of insulin. This is the kind of *diabetes* occurs most frequently in overweight adults. The disease usually can be controlled by weight loss, following a diabetic diet, and oral medications that lower blood sugar. If good sugar control can't be achieved by these methods, the use of insulin is necessary.

**Non-Hodgkin's disease.** See *lymphoma.*

**Nonprescription medication.** A medication that does not require a prescription from a doctor to obtain. This kind of medication is also referred to as over-the-counter medication because the pharmacist does not keep it locked up behind a counter. Certain antihistamines, antibiotic ointments, and mild pain killers are examples of this kind of medication.

**Non-small cell cancer.** This usually refers to the most common type of *lung cancer.* This type of lung cancer grows more slowly and is less aggressive than small cell lung cancer. However, lung cancer is the leading cause of cancer death in the United States. Most people die within five years of being diagnosed with lung cancer. Cigarette advertisements on television were outlawed because it was felt they encouraged young people to smoke and thus increased their risk of developing this and other cancers.

**Normal value.** A value or range of values considered not to indicate the presence of disease. However, all test results are subject to medical interpretation. In certain circumstances, test results may fall within the normal range of values when disease is present.

**Norwalk virus.** A virus known to be a common cause of diarrhea in adults. Symptoms usually last from twenty-four to forty-eight hours. No treatment other than maintaining proper hydration is usually required.

**Nuclear imaging.** Any imaging procedure that involves using a radioactive tracer. The tracer, usually a radioactive isotope, is injected into the body or inhaled. The dose of radiation required for the test is minimal.

**Obstetrician.** A doctor who treats women during the period of time surrounding a pregnancy and is a specialist in conditions associated with pregnancy.

**Orifice.** The entrance or exit of any part of the body.

**Osler, Sir William.** A famous physician born in Canada who lived from 1849–1919. He was an influential teacher of medicine. He published extensively and made contributions to many clinical fields of medicine.

**Osteoporosis.** A condition where bone mass has been lost, resulting in bones that aren't as strong. Some loss of bone is normal with aging in both men and women. Regular weight-bearing exercise combined with eating foods rich in calcium can help prevent osteoporosis.

**Osteosarcoma.** A *cancer* that starts in the bone. This kind of cancer usually occurs in children during their growth spurt. The most common symptom is pain.

**Out-of-network provider.** A doctor or other healthcare provider that does not participate in the health insurance plan of the patient but is providing care to the patient. Health plans do not like members to see out-of-network providers because the provider has not agreed to accept a discounted professional fee.

**Ova.** A medical word for egg.

**Over-the-counter medication.** See *nonprescription medication.*

**Packed cell volume.** See *hematocrit.*

**Pap smear.** A test used to screen for cervical *cancer*. The best time of the month to schedule a Pap smear is about two weeks after the start of a menstrual period. It is important to make sure you get the results of this test. Don't assume it is normal if you don't hear back from the doctor.

**Past medical history.** A part of the medical history that focuses on illness you have or have had in the past. It is important to go over your past problems with your doctor because they can impact your future health. For example, a past medical history of multiple sexually transmitted infections gives a doctor important information about the possible cause of infertility.

**Pathologist.** A doctor specially trained in the recognition of disease by the appearance of tissue and cells when closely examined by a microscope and other means.

**PDQ.** An independent review panel of experts selected by the National Cancer Institute. It also refers to an extensive database containing the latest information on *cancer* diagnosis, treatment, and prevention.

**Pediatric cancer center.** A medical center or section of a hospital that specializes in the treatment of *cancer* in children.

**Pediatrician.** A doctor who specializes in the treatment of children.

**Penis.** The male organ for sex and urination.

**Periodontal disease.** A disease of the structures and tissues that support the teeth. It is a common cause of tooth loss in adults. The most common symptom is bleeding gums. Good oral hygiene, regular flossing and brushing, and regular visits to the dentist can prevent this disease.

**Peripheral smear.** A blood test that gives information about the shape, number, and type of cells in the blood. Blood is smeared on a slide and examined under magnification. This can be done by a doctor, a laboratory technician, or by a machine.

**PET scan.** An abbreviation for positive emission tomography. This is an imaging technique that uses radioactive substances or tracers to distinguish normal from abnormal structures.

**Phenylketonuria.** A congenital disease that involves the failure of the amino acid phenylalanine to be metabolized properly. If not caught in infancy and treated with a low protein diet, it can result in severe mental retardation. Newborns are tested for this disease when they are born in a hospital.

**Physical examination.** A thorough examination of the body or a part of the body by a healthcare provider. A complete physical examination may include a pelvic and/or rectal examination.

**Physical signs.** A change in the body that signals illness. Physical signs are objective findings on physical examination as opposed to the subjective findings from taking a complete history of the present illness.

**Phytochemical.** A plant chemical that scientists feel may be good for your health. For example, it is believed that the carotenoids found in brightly colored fruits and vegetables may help protect against *cancer.*

**Placenta.** An organ created during pregnancy by the mother to transfer oxygen and food to the baby and remove waste materials from the baby. Normally, the placenta comes out of the womb after delivery of the baby as part of the afterbirth.

**Plague.** A contagious disease that spreads to a large area and has a high death rate. The bubonic plague and the black plague are well known examples from the history books.

**Platelets.** A component of the blood responsible for blood coagulation or clotting. When a small blood vessel is injured, platelets stick to the edges of the injury and to each other to form a patch which starts the coagulation process.

**Polyp.** A mass with a stem. When found in the colon or rectum, certain polyps can lead to *cancer.* Polyps that are known to be precancerous should be removed. This can be accomplished at time of colonoscopy and is one of the advantages of that procedure in screening for *colorectal cancer.*

**Polyunsaturated fat.** A term used to describe a type of fat. In chemistry fats are compounds composed of fatty acids. When the fatty acid contains more than one double bond between carbon atoms, it is polyunsaturated. Sunflower and safflower oils contain polyunsaturated fat.

**Potassium.** An *electrolyte* in the blood. High levels can seriously affect the heart. Normally the kidneys remove extra potassium, so high levels can be a sign of kidney trouble or use of medication that affects kidney function.

**Potassium hydroxide.** A chemical used to help detect vaginitis caused by a yeast organism.

**Prenatal care.** The medical care of the mother and baby that occurs before birth. It is important to start prenatal care early in a pregnancy to give your baby the best chance of being born healthy.

**Prescription.** A written, verbal, or electronic order for dispensing and taking a drug. It should be signed by a healthcare provider licensed to prescribe that medication. Not all doctors are licensed to prescribe strong pain drugs such as narcotics.

**Prescription medication.** A medication that can only legally be obtained with a prescription from a licensed healthcare provider.

**Primary care physician.** A physician who is trained in initial and continuing care for patients having any health concern. It includes all aspects of medicine from wellness promotion to terminal care. Part of primary care is managing the use of other health professionals and coordinating healthcare services.

**Progesterone.** A hormone produced by the ovary and the *placenta* that prepares the uterus for pregnancy. It is given along with *estrogen* in hormonal replacement therapy to women who still have a uterus because of concerns about cancer of the uterus.

**Prognosis.** An educated guess about the course of a disease.

**Prostate gland.** A gland in men that secretes seminal fluid. It can be palpated by digital rectal exam. The normal-sized prostate weighs about 20 grams.

**Prostate specific antigen (PSA).** An *antigen* released into the blood when the architecture of the prostate gland is disrupted by infection or *cancer.* A high level of PSA does not necessarily mean cancer is present in the prostate gland.

**Pulse.** The motion created by the blood as it is pumped through an artery. Taking a pulse is an easy way to determine if the heart is beating. In adults a normal pulse is between 60 to 100 beats per minute.

**Pulse oximeter.** A machine that measures the amount of oxygen in the blood. It is usually attached to the tip of a finger.

**Radiation.** Ionizing rays. In medicine these are used to obtain images of the body and to treat certain diseases.

**Radon.** A radioactive gas that occurs naturally in the soil and rocks formed by the breakdown of radium.

**RBC.** See *red blood cell.*

**RBC screen.** A test that looks at the color, size, and shape of the *red blood cells.* The results are used to help determine the cause of an *anemia.*

**Recovery period.** The time it takes to get back to normal after an illness, accident, or other event. This period is also known as convalescence.

**Rectum.** The last segment of the large intestine. It connects with the anal opening.

**Red blood cell (RBC).** A cell in the blood whose primary function is to transport oxygen to the cells of the body. The red blood cells carry *hemoglobin,* which is oxygenated in the lungs and transported by the arteries to the tissues where it is released by the capillaries. The average life span of a red blood cell is 120 days.

**Reference range.** A range of values for a test that represent the average results of tests from people free of disease.

**Respiration rate.** The number of times you inhale per unit of time. This is a measurement of how fast you are breathing.

**Reticulocyte.** An immature form of a *red blood cell.* The number of these cells in the blood increases when the bone marrow increases production of red blood cells.

**Rhesus factor.** A factor in the blood responsible for the Rh typing of the blood. You are either Rh positive or Rh negative. Mothers who are negative and who have a positive baby need to be given shots of the drug RhoGam during pregnancy to prevent sensitization and an incompatibility reaction.

**Rheumatic fever.** A disease resulting from an infection with Group A beta hemolytic streptococcus. It is believed to be an autoimmune response to an untreated infection with this bacterium. It is important to take *all* your medication when diagnosed with strep throat to prevent this complication.

**RhoGam.** A medication used to prevent Rh type blood incompatibility reactions. It is an immune globulin given during and around pregnancy.

**Risk factor.** Any factor that increases the odds of someone developing a disease or condition. Having a risk factor only increases your chances of developing a disease, it does not mean that you will definitely get the disease. However, if you have a preventable risk factor for a disease, such as smoking, you should change your behavior to eliminate the risk.

**Rotavirus.** A group of viruses that causes severe *diarrhea* in young children. Peak season for this illness, which is spread by fecal–oral transmission, is October through May.

**Rounds.** A term used to describe when a healthcare provider is providing medical care for any of his institutionalized patients. Usually this is a hospital but rounds are also made at nursing homes and other long- and short-term care facilities.

**Routine appointment.** An appointment that is scheduled at the convenience of both the patient and the healthcare provider. No medical harm will likely occur if this type of the appointment does not occur within a few days.

**RPR.** A screening test used to detect the sexually transmitted infection *syphilis*. A positive test doesn't always mean you currently are infected with the disease.

**Sarcoma.** A type of *cancer* that originates in the supportive or connective *tissues* such as bone, cartilage, or muscle.

**Saturated fat.** A term used to describe a type of fat. In chemistry fats are compounds composed of fatty acids. When the fatty acid contains a single bond between carbon atoms, it is saturated. Most saturated fats, such as butter, are pretty solid at room temperature. Although they taste great, you should limit the amount of saturated fats in your diet.

**Screening test.** A test that looks for the presence of disease when no symptoms are present. The purpose of a screening test is to recognize a disease before it has advanced to the stage where it causes symptoms. Screening is performed for diseases where early recognition and treatment have been shown to make a difference.

**Search engine.** A tool used to find Web sites related to a particular topic.

**Sed rate.** See *erythrocyte sedimentation rate.*

**Semen.** The fluid released by a male during ejaculation. In addition to fluid from the *prostate gland,* it normally contains sperm from the testicles. No sperm will be found in the semen of men who have had a vasectomy or are infertile for another reason.

**Seroconversion.** When a blood test for a disease becomes positive.

It can take up to six months for seroconversion to take place after exposure to *HIV*.

**Serum Aminotransferases.** Specific *enzymes* that act as indicators of liver injury or disease.

**Serum Glutamate Pyruvate Transaminase (SGPT).** See *ALT*.

**Serum Glutamic Oxaloacetic Transaminase (SGOT).** See *AST*.

**Sickle Cell anemia.** An inherited disease of the blood that causes chronic *anemia*. The disease affects the shape of the *red blood cells*. Instead of being disc-shaped, the cells are crescent, or sickle, shaped. This causes them to be more fragile and to break down. More common in blacks, the disease is marked by medically serious and painful episodes.

**SIDS.** See *sudden infant death syndrome*.

**Sigmoid colon.** A part of the large intestine that lies between the descending colon and the rectum.

**Sleep apnea.** A condition that results in a temporary lapse in breathing while sleeping. The partner of the patient is often the first to notice the irregular breathing pattern. It can lead to serious daytime drowsiness.

**Small cell cancer.** Usually refers to an aggressive, fast growing type of *lung cancer*.

**Smallpox.** A contagious viral disease that is thought to have been eradicated in the world. It has come to recent attention because of the threat of bioterrorism. *Vaccination* against this disease is possible.

**Sodium.** A positive ion in the blood. The amount of sodium in the blood is primarily determined by the amount eaten and the amount excreted by the kidney. The control of sodium and water are interrelated—water retention often follows sodium retention.

**Specialist.** A physician who specializes in a field of medicine such as *family practice*, obstetrics, surgery, or neurology.

**SPECT scan.** An abbreviation for single photon emission computed tomography. It is a type of imaging that uses a radioactive substance or tracer to distinguish normal from abnormal tissues.

**SPF.** Sun protective factor. Use a sun block that has an SPF rating of at least 15. Products with this level of protection will block 93 percent of burning rays.

**Stethoscope.** An instrument used to listen to the heart.

**Stool culture.** A culture performed on stool that encourages abnormal organisms in the stool to grow. It is usually ordered to find out the cause of persistent *diarrhea.*

**Stool for BOP.** A laboratory test that is performed on a sample of stool looking for blood, eggs, or parasites. It is usually performed to find out the cause of *diarrhea.*

**Strep.** A common term for the streptococcus bacteria.

**Strep throat.** A type of infection in the back of the throat caused by the streptococcus bacteria.

**Stroke.** A sudden loss of brain function caused by damage to a blood vessel in the brain. The most common cause of a stroke is *atherosclerosis.*

**Sudden Infant Death Syndrome.** The sudden death of an infant from no apparent cause. Most of these deaths occur before six months of age. It is believed that breast feeding and placing infants to sleep on their backs help prevent this syndrome.

**Suicide.** Taking one's own life.

**Sunscreen.** A product designed to help protect against ultraviolet rays from the sun. Of course, the best protection against the damaging effects of the sun is to limit exposure.

**Sympathetic nervous system.** A part of the *autonomic nervous system.* Sympathetic effects tend to be general in nature and help the body deal with stressful situations.

**Symptom.** A change in the body or normal functions noticed by a patient that can signal disease.

**Syphilis.** A specific sexually transmitted infection. The first sign of the disease is a small painless ulceration called a *chancre.* The disease can be cured by antibiotics.

**Systolic blood pressure.** The top number of a *blood pressure* reading. This is the pressure that occurs with contraction of the ventricles of the heart.

**Testosterone.** The male sex hormone. It is produced by the testes and is responsible for the development of masculine characteristics. A synthetic version is available to treat deficiencies of this hormone.

**Tetanus.** A life-threatening illness caused by a toxin from the bacteria *Clostridium tetani.* Typically this occurs when a wound becomes contaminated by this organism. The disease can be prevented with *immunization.*

**Thin prep.** A technique where sample cervical cells are suspended in a liquid rather than spread on a slide and sent to a laboratory to screen for cervical cancer. This process is a newer way to perform a *Pap smear.*

**Total cholesterol.** The total amount of *cholesterol* in the blood. This is the sum of the HDL and LDL levels. Normal cholesterol is currently considered to be less than 200mg/dl.

**Total protein.** The amount of protein in the blood. This laboratory test indicates nutritional status of the body as well as kidney and liver function.

**Toxoplasmosis.** Usually a mild febrile illnesses caused by a parasite that thrives in cats. One of the ways to contract the illness is by handling infected cat feces. The illness can have serious consequences for pregnant women and people with a compromised immune system.

**Triage.** A way to sort patients by the acuteness of their need for medical attention.

**Triglyceride.** A type of fat in the blood. High levels are associated with heart disease.

**Trust-e.** This is a nonprofit organization that is concerned with protecting the privacy of personal medical information on the Internet.

**Trustmark.** A seal Web sites that meet the privacy standards set by Trust-e are allowed to display.

**Tularemia.** A disease transmitted to humans by infected bugs and animals. Attention has been brought to this disease by the threat of bioterrorism.

**Type 1 diabetes.** See *IDDM.*

**Type 2 diabetes.** See *NIDDM.*

**Ultrasound.** An imaging technique that uses high frequency sound waves to create a picture.

**United States Preventive Services Task Force (USPSTF).** A task force with members representing all specialties of medicine. It reviews medical research and makes recommendations for standards of medical practice. For example, this task force is responsible for setting the standards for medical disease screening.

**URAC.** See *American Accreditation Healthcare Commission.*

**Urethra.** The tube that goes from the bladder to the outside of the body. When you urinate, the urine comes out of your urethra.

**Urinalysis.** A laboratory test where a technician, doctor, or other healthcare provider looks at substances contained in the urine. In the doctor's office this is usually accomplished with a dip stick.

**URL.** The address of a Web site.

**USPSTF.** See *United States Preventive Services Task Force.*

**Vaccine.** A suspension containing material designed to stimulate an immune response and protect against disease. It can be given as a shot, swallowed, or sprayed into the nose.

**Vaccination.** An inoculation with a vaccine.

**Vagina.** The mucous membrane-lined canal between the cervix and the vulva in a female.

**Vaginitis.** An infection of the vaginal canal.

**Viagra.** A drug made by Pfizer used to treat male impotence.

**Viral hemorrhagic fevers.** A class of viral illnesses of varying severity. Recent attention has been brought to these diseases as a result of the threat of bioterrorism.

**Vital signs.** A person's pulse, respirations, blood pressure, and temperature. These are physical findings concerning the functions vital to life. Some healthcare providers consider pain a vital sign, but unlike the others it can't be objectively measured.

**Wave scheduling.** An appointment scheduling technique that takes into account the way patients flow into the office under normal conditions.

**Weight.** In medical terms, the force of gravity on your body. Your ideal weight is the number of pounds you should weigh based upon your height and frame to achieve or maintain the best health.

**Wet prep.** A test that looks at discharge obtained from the vagina to find the source of an infection.

**White blood cell (WBC).** There are five types of white blood cells: *neutrophils, eosinophils, basophils, lymphocytes,* and *monocytes.* The first three are also called granulocytes. White blood cells help the body fight infection.

**White blood count.** A test that measures the number of *white blood cells.* White blood cells help the body fight off disease. White blood cell counts may be high with bacterial infections.

**White cell morphology.** This test looks at the different types of white cells in the blood. In addition to estimating the percentage of each type of cell present, this test also notes any cells that appear abnormal in color, shape, or size. This test is also known as a differential or a peripheral smear.

**Wilm's tumor.** A type of kidney *cancer* that occurs in children. It is thought to arise from fetal kidney tissue although the exact cause is unknown.

**X-ray.** A form of imaging where radiation is passed through the body to create a picture. Dense parts of the body block most of the rays and appear whiter on the film than more absorbent tissues.

# NOTES

## CHAPTER 1: THE TYPICAL OFFICE VISIT

1. G. D. Lundberg with J. Stacy, *Severed Trust: Why American Medicine Has Not Been Fixed* (New York: Basic Books, 2001).

2. Ibid.

## CHAPTER 2: HOW DOCTORS MAKE A DIAGNOSIS

1. P. G. Ramsey, J. R. Curtis, and D. S. Paauw, "History-Taking and Preventive Medicine Skills among Primary Care Physicians: An Assessment Using Standardized Patients," *American Journal of Medicine* 104, no. 2 (February 1998): 152–58.

2. R. Mittendorf et al., "Strenuous Physical Activity in Young Adulthood and Risk of Breast Cancer (United States)," *Cancer Causes Control* 6, no. 4 (July 1995): 347–53; C. E. Matthews et al., "Lifetime Physical Activity and Breast Cancer Risk in the Shanghai Breast Cancer Study," *British Journal of Cancer* 84, no. 7 (April 6, 2001): 994–1001.

## CHAPTER 3: HOW TO WORK WITH YOUR DOCTOR

1. J. Y. Reginster et al., "Long Term Effects of Glucosamine Sulfate on Osteoarthritis Progression: A Randomised, Placebo-Controlled Clinical Trial," *The Lancet* 357 (2001): 251–56.
2. M. H. Schien et al., "Treating Hypertension with a Device That Slows and Regularises Breathing: A Randomised, Double-Blind Controlled Study," *Journal of Human Hypertension* 15 (2001): 271–78.


## CHAPTER 4: GOOD HEALTH AT EVERY STAGE OF LIFE

1. National Center for Health Statistics, "Relationship of Cancer to the Leading Causes of Death in the United States" [online], www.nci.nih.gov/public/factbk95/crelate.htm.
2. *National Vital Statistics Report* 49, no. 12 (October 9, 2001): 25–26.
3. Ibid.
4. Ibid.
5. Ibid.
6. Ibid.
7. National Center for Health Statistics, "Relationship of Cancer."
8. J. Reed and N. Shulman, *The Black Man's Guide to Good Health* (Roscoe, Ill.: Hilton Publishing, 2001).
9. *National Vital Statistics Report.*


## CHAPTER 5: HOW TO AVOID ILLNESS

1. D. Pittet et al., "Effectiveness of a Hospital-Wide Programme to Improve Compliance with Hand Hygiene Infection Control Programme," *Lancet* 356 (2000): 1307–12.
2. L. Roberts, "Effects of Infection Control Measures on the Frequency of Diarrheal Episodes in Child Care: A Randomized, Controlled Trial," *Pediatrics* 105 (April 1, 2000): 743–46; M. E. Guinan, M. McGuckin-Guinan, and A. Sevareid, "Who Washes Hands after Using the Bathroom?" *American Journal of Infection Control* 25 (October 1997): 424–25.
3. M. K. Ryan, R. Christian, and J. Wohlrahe, "Handwashing to

Reduce Illness among Young Adults in Navy Recuit Training," *Naval Health Recruiting Center Publication* 99–18.

4. M. Berthold, "Oral-Systemic Links" [online], www.ada.org [accessed September 17, 2001].

5. F. Pentimone and L. Del Corso, "Why Regular Physical Actvity Favors Longevity," *Minerva Medicine* 89 (June 1998): 197–201.

6. S. A. New, "Current Issues Concerning Optimum Nutrition and Health Outcomes" [online] www.medscape.com [*Medscape Women's Health* 6, no. 4 (2001)].

7. A. Taylor, P. F. Jacques, E. M. Epstein, "Relations among Aging, Antioxidant Status, and Cataract," *American Journal of Clinical Nutrition* 62 suppl 6 (December 1995): 1439S–1447S; M. Seddon et al., "Dietary Carotenoids, Vitamins A, C, and E, and Advanced Age-Related Macular Degeneration," *Journal of the American Medical Association* 272 (November 9, 1994): 1413–20.

8. A. J. Perkins et al., "Association of Antioxidants with Memory in a Multiethnic Elderly Sample Using the Third National Health and Nutrition Examination Survey," *American Journal of Epidemiology* 150 (1999): 37–44.

9. Y. Wan et al., "Effects of Cocoa Powder and Dark Chocolate on LDL Oxidative Susceptibility and Prostaglandin Concentrations in Humans," *American Journal of Clinical Nutrition* 74 (November 2001): 596–602.

10. "Food Safety in Restaurants," *Healthy Lifestyles* [online] www.healthatoz.com [accessed November 13, 2001].

11. "Vaccine Information Database," *National Network for Immunization Information* [online] www.immunoizationinfo.org; "Vaccine Information Statements," *Centers for Disease Control* [online] www.cdc.gov/nip.

12. American Academy of Family Physicians, "2001AAFP Clinical Recommendations"; "The Third U.S. Preventive Services Task Force: Background, Methods, and First Recommendations," *American Journal of Preventive Medicine* 20, suppl 3 (2001).

13. American Association of Clinical Endocrinologists, "Press Release" August 2001.

14. G. L. Carlo and R. S. Jenrow, "Scientific Progress–Wireless Phones and Brain Cancer: Current State of the Science," *Medscape* [online] www.medscape.com [MedGenMed, July 31, 2000].

15. J. B. Laundzen, M. M. Peterson, and B. Lund, "Effect of External Hip Protectors on Hip Fractures," *Lancet* 341 (January 2, 1993).

16. L. J. Horwood, "Breastfeeding and Later Cognitive and Academic Outcomes," *Pediatrics* 101, E9 (January 1, 1998).

17. "Rx for a Better Life? Get a Pet, and Do It Now" [online] rev.tamu.edu/stories/01/110101-2.html; S. K. Wong, L. H. Feinstein, and P. Heidman, "Healthy Pets, Healthy People," *Journal of American Veterinary Medicine* 215 (August 1, 1999): 335–38.

18. G. Anandarajah and E. Hight, "Spirituality and Medical Practice: Using the HOPE Questions as a Practical Tool for Spiritual Assessment," *American Family Practitioner* (January 2001): 81–89.

## CHAPTER 6: UNDERSTANDING YOUR MEDICAL TEST RESULTS

1. Rakel, *Conn's Current Therapy 2001*, 53rd ed. (Philadelphia: W. B. Saunders Company, 2001) [online] www.mdconsult.com.
2. Ibid.
3. Ibid.
4. Ibid.
5. Ibid.
6. Ibid.
7. Ibid.
8. Ibid.
9. Ibid.
10. Ibid.
11. Ibid.
12. Ibid.
13. Ibid.
14. Ibid.
15. Ibid.
16. Ibid.
17. Ibid.
18. "Product information" [online] www.givenimaging.com.

## CHAPTER 7: INTERNET SOURCES OF QUALITY HEALTH INFORMATION AND CARE

1. G. D. Lundberg with J. Stacy, *Severed Trust: Why American Medicine Has Not Been Fixed* (New York: Basic Books, 2001), p. 131.

# BIBLIOGRAPHY

Berhman, *Nelson Textbook of Pediatrics*, 16th ed. (Philadelphia: W. B. Saunders Company, 2000) [online] www.mdconsult.com.

*Brenner and Rector's The Kidney*, 6th ed. (Philadelphia: W. B. Saunders Company, 2000) [online] www.mdconsult.com.

*Clinician's Handbook of Preventive Services*, 2nd ed. (ACHR1998) [online] www.ahcpr.gov/clinic/ppiphand.htm.

Goetz, *Textbook of Clinical Neurology* (Philadelphia: W. B. Saunders Company, 1999) [online] www.mdconsult.com.

Goldman, *Cecil's Textbook of Medicine*, 21st ed. (Philadelphia: W. B. Saunders Company, 2000) [online] www.mdconsult.com.

Goroll, *Primary Care Medicine*, 4th ed. (Philadelphia: Lippincott Williams and Wilkens, 2000) [online] www.mdconsult.com.

Juhl, *Paul and Juhl's Essentials of Radiologic Imaging*, 7th ed. (Philadelphia: Lippincott Williams and Wilkens, 1998) [online] www.mdconsult.com.

Lee, *Wintrobe's Clinical Hematology*, 10th ed. (Philadelphia: Lippincott Williams and Wilkens, 1999) [online] www.mdconsult.com.

Mandell, *Principles and Practice of Infectious Disease*, 5th ed. (New York: Churchhill Livingstone, Inc., 2000) [online] www.mdconsult.com.

"Medical Management of Bioterror, Excerpted from USAMRIID's Medical Management of Biological Casualties Handbook," [online] www.medexact.com.

Noble, *Textbook of Primary Care Medicine*, 3rd ed. (St. Louis, Mo.: Mosby, Inc., 2001) [online] www.mdconsult.com.

Pizzo and Poplack, *Principles and Practice of Pediatric Onocology*, 3rd ed. (Philadelphia: Lippincott-Raven Publishers, 1997) [online] www.mdconsult.com.

Rakel, *Conn's Current Therapy 2001*, 53rd ed. (Philadelphia: W. B. Saunders Company, 2001) [online] www.mdconsult.com.

Ravel, *Clinical Laboratory Medicine*, 6th ed. (St. Louis, Mo.: Mosby-Year Book, Inc., 1995) [online] www.mdconsult.com.

*Taber's Electronic Cyclopedic Medical Dictionary vs 2.0* (Philadelphia: F. A. Davis Co., 2001) [online] www.tabers.com.

# INDEX

saturated fat, 96, 110, 143, 144, 275
schedule, 28, 29, 30, 31, 33, 37, 41, 50, 59, 101, 118, 140, 249, 270
semen, 87, 104, 275
seroconversion, 90, 276
SGOT. *See* AST.
SGPT. *See* ALT.
sickle cell anemia, 77, 78, 172. *See also* hemoglobinopathy.
side effect, 40, 68, 85, 104, 107, 110, 179, 215
sigmoid colon, 97, 251
sleep apnea, 139
small cell cancer. *See* lung cancer.
smallpox, 127, 276
sodium, 176, 178, 181, 191, 250, 255, 276
specialist, 24, 25, 26, 58, 70, 270
stethoscope, 35, 75
stool BOP, 194
stool culture, 194
stroke, 109, 111, 113, 115, 116, 122, 143, 173, 177–79, 218, 247, 250, 264, 266, 268, 277
sudden infant death syndrome (SIDS), 73, 78, 79, 276
suicide, 84, 85, 230
sunscreen, 159, 160
sympathetic nervous system. *See* autonomic nervous system.
syphilis, 89, 188, 250, 257, 275
systolic blood pressure. *See* blood pressure.

testosterone, 66, 67, 237
tetanus, 65, 67, 151, 154, 155
thyroid stimulating hormone, 184

total cholesterol, 110, 179
total protein, 183
triage, 30
triglycerides, 158
Trust-e, 278
Tularemia, 278
Type 1 diabetes. *See* diabetes mellitis.
Type 2 diabetes. *See* diabetes mellitis.

ultrasound, 102, 107, 196, 199
United States National Center for Health Statistics, 73
United States Preventive Services Task Force, 34, 96, 100, 106, 157, 192, 278, 279
unsaturated fat, 143
URAC. *See* American Accreditation Healthcare Commission.

vaccine, 87, 120, 126, 128, 150, 152, 153, 155, 264, 279
Viagra, 104, 279
viral hemorrhagic fevers, 128

Wet prep, 279
white blood count, 169, 173, 265, 280
white cell morphology. *See* leukocyte count.
Wilm's Tumor, 81, 280

X-ray, 56, 58, 92, 97, 100–101, 119, 196–99, 248, 251–52, 256, 266–67, 280